Praise for *Yoga for Life*

"Colleen tells her story and how yoga has unraveled the knots that have been stored from different traumas and everyday life. The yoga solutions she offers are a first aid kit. This book is a must for your library of home health."

—Mark Hyman, MD, director, Cleveland Clinic Center for Functional Medicine, and author of *The Blood Sugar Solution 10-Day Detox Diet*

"Colleen Saidman Yee's life has been a wild ride that, thankfully, led her to yoga. Her story, her insights, and her yoga sequences will improve your emotional, physical, and mental well-being, and help you onto the path of peace and freedom."

—Frank Lipman, MD, author of *Revive*

"Colleen inspires me as a woman, a mother, and a girlfriend, always coming from a place of love and kindness. Her teaching is that yoga is as simple as a breath. Reading her book is like having a woman-to-woman conversation with an honest, nurturing, and encouraging friend who shares and cares with all her heart. It is a powerful wake-up call to the spirit within, with real down-to-earth strategies to empower yourself through this beautiful journey called life."

—Donna Karan, founder and chief designer of Donna Karan New York and Urban Zen

"Here in *Yoga for Life* are fantastic instructions and sequences for feeling and releasing the stories and games that bind us. Colleen's confessions and experiences teach a compassionate embrace of the shadow. I highly recommend her book to anyone wanting to be free."

—Richard Freeman, author of *The Mirror of Yoga*

"Like Gandhi, Colleen is *satyagraha*—meaning possessed by the truth. She tells her story honestly, without pretense, no makeup—totally fearless while at the same time gracefully imbuing every word with infectious joy, gratitude, and compassion. You will find no blaming or complaining in this memoir, for this is the story of a remarkable woman who approaches life as an adventure, armed with a bewitching ability to transform obstacles into opportunities and the ordinary into something magical. She is living proof that yoga is for life."

—Sharon Gannon, Jivamukti Yoga

"Colleen is a strong, empowering woman who I look to for sisterhood and wisdom. She has used every crazy twist and turn of her own life to find her spiritual center, and now she teaches us how to do the same. Her unfiltered honesty will break you open and give you courage to find personal freedom as you reevaluate your own stories. Colleen's funny, moving, and compassionate approach helps women set down their shame and pick up their voices. Her work has helped me to find more joy and contentment through asana, honest self-reflection, and loving-kindness. This book is a treasure."

—Kris Carr, author of *Crazy Sexy Cancer Tips*

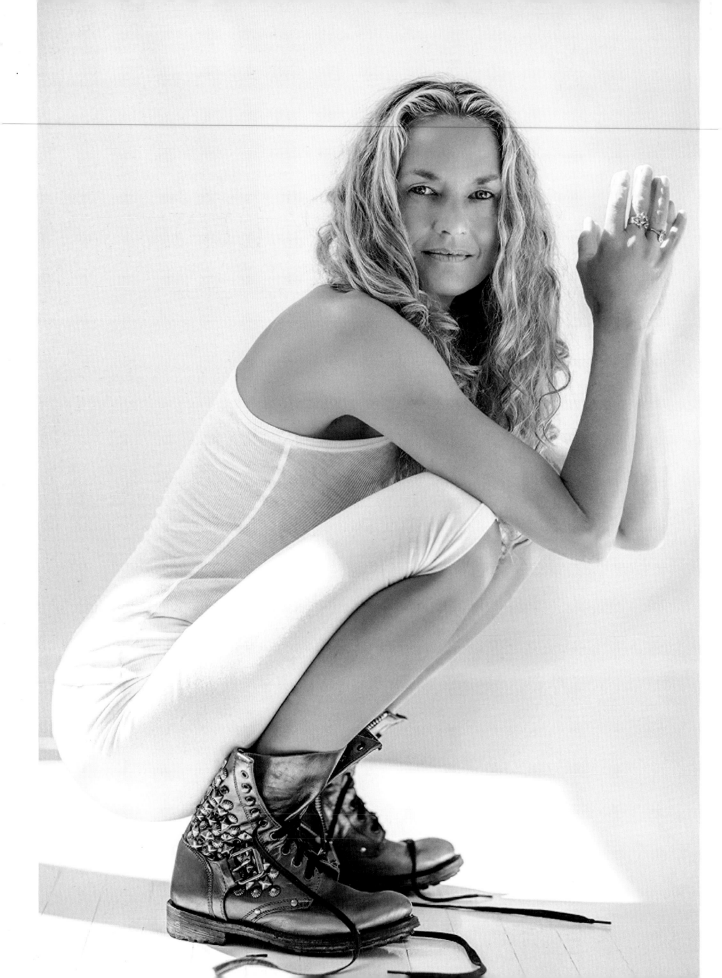

YOGA FOR LIFE

A JOURNEY TO INNER PEACE AND FREEDOM

COLLEEN SAIDMAN YEE

with Susan K. Reed

Afterword by Rodney Yee

ATRIA PAPERBACK

NEW YORK · LONDON · TORONTO · SYDNEY · NEW DELHI

ATRIA PAPERBACK

An Imprint of Simon & Schuster, Inc.
1230 Avenue of the Americas
New York, NY 10020

First Atria Paperback edition June 2015

ATRIA PAPERBACK and colophon are trademarks of Simon & Schuster, Inc.

For information about special discounts for bulk purchases, please contact Simon & Schuster Special Sales at 1-866-506-1949 or business@simonandschuster.com.

The Simon & Schuster Speakers Bureau can bring authors to your live event. For more information or to book an event contact the Simon & Schuster Speakers Bureau at 1-866-248-3049 or visit our website at www.simonspeakers.com.

Interior design by Paul Dippolito

Manufactured in the United States of America

10 9 8 7 6 5 4 3 2 1

Library of Congress Cataloging-in-Publication Data

Saidman Yee, Colleen.
  Yoga for life : a journey to inner peace and freedom / Colleen Saidman Yee, with Susan K. Reed.
— First [edition].
     pages cm
  Includes index.
  Saidman Yee, Colleen. 2. Yogis—United States—Biography. I. Title.
  B132.Y6S36365 2015
  613.7'046092—dc23
  [B]
                                      2014045823
ISBN 978-1-4767-7678-1
ISBN 978-1-4767-7680-4 (ebook)

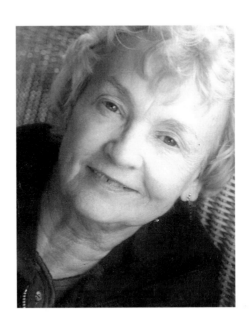

I dedicate this book to the strong, feisty Irishwoman
who showed me what love is.
I miss you, Mom.

What would happen if one woman told the truth about her life?
The world would split open.

—"KATHE KOLLWITZ," MURIEL RUKEYSER

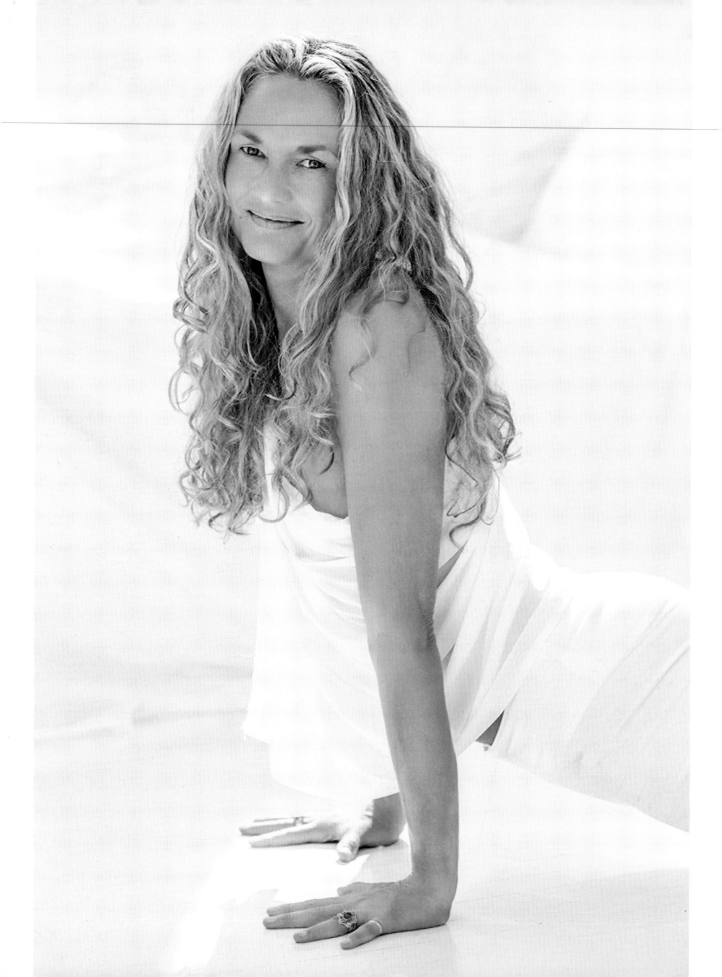

CONTENTS

INTRODUCTION:
KNOW YOU'RE ENOUGH

I watch women's chests. I watch the arches of their feet. I watch the positions of their pelvises and the placement of their heads. I watch women holding it all together, afraid that if they slow down, everything will fall apart. I watch women being ashamed that they are aging and feeling unworthy of love. I watch women collapse.

I also watch women's perfection, courage, compassion, and grace. We women can balance our heads over our lifted chests, supported by strong legs that are connected to the earth. We can raise the arches of our feet and we can soften our faces. We can carry ourselves in the world with confidence and ease.

I've taught yoga to thousands of women (and men) for close to two decades. Women are powerful and beautiful, and we are also in pain—physical, emotional, and psychological—stemming from past or present trauma. We're fearful about what the future may or may not bring, personally or professionally. Women in my classes cope with addiction, body and relationship issues, mother issues, competitiveness, and an inability to tell the truth. All of these things create stagnation and tension in the body. Yoga gives us tools to overcome the obstacles that exist between us and freedom, joy, and gratitude. I see why women come to yoga; they want to reclaim something in themselves. It's inspiring to watch women gain a different perspective and fall in love with their bodies.

I was a professional model for three decades and very confused about my value beyond my looks. I've experienced triumphs in life, but plenty of traumas, too. I've always been searching for something beyond what I can see, hear, smell, taste, and touch. I've had glimpses of this mystery through prayer, intense exercise, and drugs. Yet it is yoga that takes me back to myself and has made me realize that the magic that I've spent my lifetime searching for is right here inside of me. All I have to do is stop running from it.

My yoga journey started in 1987 when a friend convinced me to go with her to a yoga class in New York City. When I walked out, I felt different than I'd ever felt in my life. As I stepped into the street and its lights, colors, and smells—all seemed different, so crisp and so clear. Something significant had shifted, and something opened up inside of me. I felt alive in a whole new way.

I love this definition of yoga from one of my first teachers, Sharon Gannon: "Yoga is the state where nothing is missing." When was the last time we felt nothing was missing? Maybe in utero.

The term *satya* means "truthfulness" in Sanskrit. So many of us are lying to ourselves; we're putting an identity out there that we want other people to see, and we're hiding, from ourselves and from others, who we truly are. In truthfulness as in yoga, nothing is missing. We are present, whole.

Even after all my years of practice and study, I can't claim to know what enlightenment is, or if yoga will take me there. But I do know that yoga lowers stress, improves posture, circulation, and digestion, while keeping joints fluid and muscles toned. It may also be the best antiaging regimen we have, and it can bring us to our ideal weight. Yoga eases everyday pains and frustrations and increases kindness and compassion. It hones the body and stabilizes the mind. Yoga can illuminate our spirits and free us from the shackles of our stories, which often limit our vision of who we are and what we are capable of achieving.

When you navigate the inner landscapes of your body through breath work, mindfulness, and postures, you notice if what you have just said, done, or thought makes you feel lousy or good. One day several years ago, my four-year-old nephew, Johnny, was talking to my oldest brother, Mark. Johnny said, "Uncle Mark, I really love everyone!" Mark replied: "Really, Johnny? I don't love everyone. In fact, I even have enemies." Johnny shook his head and said, "That's too bad, Uncle Mark. You must feel so bad inside." This awareness is the first step toward right thought, right word, right action, and maybe even peace. It could be that simple.

One night, my husband, Rodney, and I were surfing YouTube videos when we stumbled on a video of a Fiona Apple concert. It was an "aha!" moment for me. I thought: *This woman is telling the truth with her body*. She's not what you would typically call a good dancer, she was jerky and unconcerned about looking pretty, but something about her was raw and real. She was moving with her wounds, with her limitations—she was moving truthfully. She wasn't hiding, and she wasn't afraid to be vulnerable and expose herself through her voice and movements.

Her courage and honesty made her dance mesmerizing and powerful. It penetrated something deep inside me. When you bow to someone and say, *"Namaste,"* it means, "The deepest part of me acknowledges the deepest part of you." Fiona Apple's performance was a *Namaste* from her body to mine. I want to have the courage to be as honest in my life, my teaching, and in this book as she was in that dance.

Yoga can bring you to this kind of truth by helping you to observe, then to let go of, the habits you cling to and the stories you use to protect yourself. As you practice, you become intimate with your body, which many of us spend a lifetime either alienated from or waging war with. Yoga practice can pierce emotional places that most of us guard or avoid. Our bodies are intelligent, more a source of direct truth than our minds, but we rarely listen to the wisdom that's buried in our beautiful chambers.

I became a yoga teacher because I have experienced the real change yoga can create. With yoga, I'm at home in my skin. Yoga has helped me to become more honest. It has helped me discover my body, and through it, my voice.

In the modern yoga world, yogis were often put into little boxes and expected to be celibate, or cult members, or tree-hugging, granola-eating hippies. I'm here to tell you that today a yogi can be anyone, even an Irish Italian girl from the heartland of Indiana.

Yoga has given me a larger family, my yoga community, a congregation of people willing to work to find the connectivity that's sometimes hidden. It brings to the surface what we need to feel and know. The late B. K. S. Iyengar, perhaps the most influential yoga teacher of our age, said that you can only be as intimate with others as you are with yourself. Alone and in community, we use yoga to get to our essence. Yoga peels away layer after layer of debris to uncover what has been there all along. It's like the Bob Dylan lyric: "How long, babe, will you search for what's not lost?"

This is the story of one woman's life, my life, in and out of yoga. It isn't always pretty, but it's as honest as I can be, and as memory allows. I've tried to extract from my journey some of the painful and exuberant lessons I've learned, and I've embodied each of them in a unique yoga sequence. For dealing with suffering, the sequences are intended to be soothing and nurturing; for dealing with growth and other life passages, the sequences are intended to be celebratory and to lead you to your own insights. The sequences I've designed address issues of alienation, addiction, and insecurity as well as finding one's voice and participating in the endless potential of acceptance and love.

The goal of a yoga sequence is to create a physical effect, an emotional effect, and a spiritual effect. The key is to investigate and listen to your body, to increase intimacy with it in order to understand cause and effect. What sequence of poses, breath work, and meditation creates greater peace? (Not just peace in our joints, but peace in our guts, our hearts, our nervous systems, and our lives.) We're all "sequencing" every day. If you need to drop the kids off at school and go to the bank, the post office, and the grocery store, you figure out an optimal order in which to complete those tasks. When it comes to the body, the same lessons apply. Yoga is skill in action; part of that skill is learning the right sequence, on and off the mat.

A beautiful yoga playground awaits you in these pages, and, I hope, the sequences I've created will reveal the blue sky that's waiting inside you.

Today, I'm fifty-five years old and happily married. I don't do drugs, and I'm a vegetarian. Instead of chasing synthetic highs, I've learned how to extract a high from the beauty of an ordinary day. I've learned that the best high exists in the joy or the sadness or the mundaneness of the present moment, unfiltered. Yoga allows me to surf the ripples and sit with the mud, all while catching glimpses of the clarity at the bottom of the lake: my true Self.

I hope this book will help you do the same. *Namaste.*

YOGA FOR LIFE

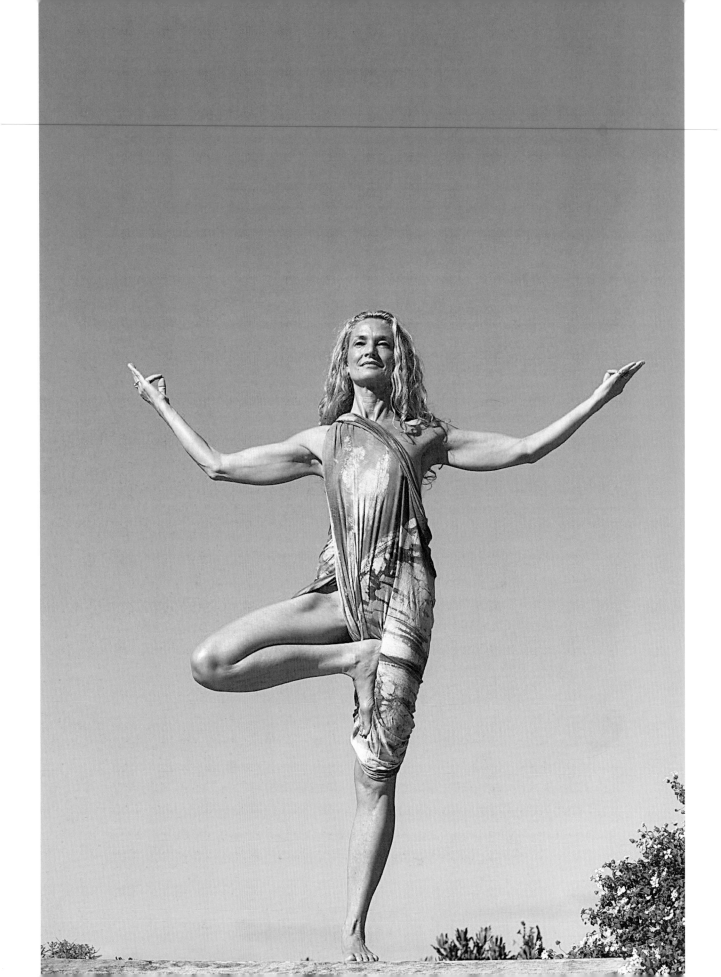

Chapter 1

ROOTS

Be still, my heart, these great trees are prayers.
—"Stray Birds," Rabindranath Tagore

A scene that's permanently etched in my brain opens in 1967 in the kitchen of a house in a new subdivision of a small farming town called Bluffton, Indiana. Our family has recently moved here from Corning, New York. There are empty moving boxes everywhere, a new playground for hide-and-seek. I crawl into one of the boxes, which easily fits my wiry seven-year-old body. I'm secretly watching my mother, who's standing across the room, looking out the window with a cup of coffee in one hand and a cigarette in the other. She seems to be in a trance, and big tears are sliding down her face like swollen raindrops. She's whispering prayers as she often does when she's alone. I'm confused. At this age, I don't think moms are supposed to cry. She's probably figured out that I've been secretly pinching my little brother Nick and stealing his toys. I'm sick of him being Mr. Goody Two-shoes. I stare at my mother helplessly, mesmerized by the smoke from her cigarette as its ash grows longer. I know that it's my job to make her happy. I'm going to be perfect.

A few days later, I ask, as nonchalantly as I can, "Mom, what makes you so sad?"

"I miss my trees," she says.

Today, as I stand at my own window with a cup of tea in my hand, gazing out at the beautiful, mature trees outside, I wish I could tell my mother that I understand her connection with trees. I realize now, that on that morning, Mom was doing her own form of yoga. She was practicing *drishti* (a soft-focused yoga gaze) out the window toward the memory of her cherished trees. She was calming herself by filling and emptying her lungs, which is like *pranayama* (yogic breathing exercises), except hers, unfortunately, involved a cigarette. She was repeating her own quiet prayer over and over. In yoga, we call this a mantra. Gaze, breath work, and mantra are ways to calm the mind in preparation for meditation. Mom's tears represented her open heart, her willingness to feel and sit with her sadness, rather than mask it. Damn, my mom was a yogi. Who knew? I'd thought yoga was my discovery, quite separate from anything she taught me.

◆　◆　◆

"*Famiglia!*" my dad would say in his fake Italian accent. "*Famiglia* is the most important thing in life. You always do what needs to be done for family." The Zello roots were in Corning, New York, where my dad, Nick, was a foreman on the swing shift at the Corning Glass Works factory. It was a grueling schedule. One week he would be on the 8:00 a.m. to 4:00 p.m. shift, the next week it was 4:00 p.m. to midnight, and the following week was the dreaded midnight to 8:00 a.m. shift, with only a day off in between. His work schedule wreaked havoc on our family life. We were always being shushed so that we wouldn't wake Dad. The days that he was

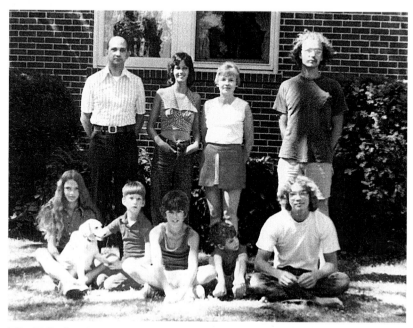

The Zello family, circa 1972: (back row, from left) Dad, Peggy, Mom, Mark; (front row, from left) me (holding our dog, Poco), Ed, Nick, John, and Joe.

able to be at the supper table with us were our happiest. Mom and Dad wanted more than anything in the world for Dad to work a regular shift so that we could spend time together as a family.

One day, Dad and Mom gathered us kids together in the living room. At the time, there were five of us: Mark, Joe, Peg, me, and Nick, in that order. Mark was fourteen, and the rest of us fell into line at approximately two-year intervals. "Guess what?" Dad announced. "We're moving to Indiana. I'm going to work in another Corning plant there. I'm going to work real hours, like other dads—nine to five!" My seven-year-old mind responded, "Oh, good! We'll be able to play during the day without Dad coming out of his bedroom yelling at us for waking him up."

We younger kids had no idea what "moving" meant, but Mark and Joe understood, and they were pissed. Today, Joe says that leaving Corning was like being dragged from a warm sleeping bag and tossed naked into a snowbank, shocking his system into angry self-defense.

The move would take us away from our beloved hometown, where *famiglia* and community were everything. In Corning, we lived across the street from St. Vincent de Paul Catholic Church and School. Our lives and Corning's Italian/Irish community revolved around St. Vincent's. When the bells pealed on Sunday, hundreds of people would surge through the big oak doors. When Mass was over, the doors would swing open again, and everyone would spill out, dressed in their Sunday best, joking and exchanging news. My brothers were altar boys (which I was jealous of) and sold newspapers after Mass.

I was a child of the Church. When I was young, I told everyone I was going to be a nun when I grew up, just like my first-grade teacher Sister Cormac. Every Halloween I would dress up as a nun. One year, my brother Joe told me that I should put a pillow under my habit and be a pregnant nun. I didn't see why not, and couldn't understand why everyone laughed at me.

My mother went to Mass almost every day and never missed confession. She always had a rosary in one hand and a cigarette in the other. I was convinced she had a direct line to Virgin Mother Mary. If Mom hadn't always been pregnant, I would have said that she was the reincarnation of Mary.

Eventually, I became disillusioned with the Catholic Church. I was brought up to believe that priests were representatives of Jesus Christ; when charges of pedophilia became rampant, I was profoundly disheartened. I also saw that the underlying doctrine, which holds that we're all sinners meant to suffer and ask for redemption, had tormented my mother and she became riddled with guilt.

In many ways, yoga became my church, even though I don't see it as a religion. Both create a community of people who gather for an hour or more of shared activity, which includes silence, listening to a teaching, reading, and chanting. The candles and incense are reminiscent of Mass. In the studio, I often play religious music such as "Ave Maria" or "Amazing Grace" as students lie in final relaxation (*shavasana*). Music brings us into the deep spaces of our own being. It's not a coincidence that I've taught yoga every Sunday morning for the last seventeen years. Our Sunday best may be Lycra, but we gather to practice and contemplate how we can be loving and caring in our everyday lives. When I plan a class, I'm usually exploring a particular topic (not unlike the subject of a homily) in the yoga sequence and in a reading at the end of class. These subjects are often related to yoga's ethical precepts (called *yamas* and *niyamas*): nonviolence, truthfulness, nonstealing, containment, nonhoarding, cleanliness, contentment, purification, self-study, and devotion.

✦   ✦   ✦

On a hot day in August 1967 we piled into our Ford Country Squire station wagon with its faux-wood side panels and started the drive to Indiana—and our new life. Dad kept stopping so that my mom could lean out the door and throw up. Mark and I looked at each other. *Uh-oh. Mom's pregnant again.* She hadn't told us, but Mark and I knew, and Mark was furious. He was old enough to see how difficult it was for my parents to pay the bills for five children on a factory worker's salary. Why the hell were they having more kids?

The Zellos rolled into Bluffton with our suitcases, household possessions—and all our emotional baggage. As one of only a handful of Italian families, we didn't fit Bluffton's prevailing ethnic type, which was German and Amish. No welcome wagons showed up to greet us. The Catholic church in Bluffton was out on the edge of town, and the congregation's size and energy were minuscule in comparison to our church in Corning.

In yoga philosophy, seeing others as separate from ourselves is thought to be one of the main causes of suffering. The Indian spiritual teacher Nisargadatta said that if you think of someone as separate from you, you won't be able to fully love them. Separation can create fear, fear deepens alienation, and alienation deepens fear in a vicious cycle. In retrospect, I think about how people in Bluffton created those separations. The Midwestern kids taunted us for pronouncing "a" differently and for the tan lines above our ankles from wearing socks with our sneakers in summer. Local boys began picking fights with my brothers—which they soon found out wasn't such a good idea. Joe is incredibly smart and can cut someone down to size with a few well-chosen words. One day, the roughest, biggest guys in town were teasing Joe, and he was mouthing off right back at them. One of the mean kids took a swing at Joe. Mark stepped in and went after him. The kid head-butted Mark and knocked out his front teeth. Mark tore the chain off the guy's motorcycle jacket and beat the crap out of the bullies with it. Let's just say the Zello boys earned some respect.

✦ ✦ ✦

Is violence ever warranted? In the *Yoga Sutras*, the first ethical precept is *ahimsa*—nonviolence or nonharming. This includes not only physical violence, but also the violence of thoughts and words. *Ahimsa* doesn't mean "pacifism"; it means we take responsibility for our own harming behaviors and we try to prevent others from causing harm. The *Bhagavad Gita*, which is a poem within the epic Hindu sacred text, the *Mahabharata*, tells the story of a warrior, Prince Arjuna, who must go into battle because it's his *dharma*—his obligation or purpose in life—to protect his people. His quandary, which he discusses with his guide, Lord Krishna, is that some of the enemies he will be forced to fight (and kill) are his relatives and teachers. Krishna tells him to buck up, that he must take action and follow through with his purpose. The important thing is that he act in a selfless spirit of sacrifice and devotion, which creates a different karmic result than if he were motivated by ego or anger.

I've always felt uncomfortable with how *Bhagavad Gita* engages the subject of violence. But I realize it has to be addressed, and there are no simple answers. If I caught someone abusing my daughter, or any child, I think I would have the potential to become violent. By acting violently, might I potentially save other children from the same fate? Sometimes violence can be a nasty look or comment. Is punching someone who is hurting a family member the same as harming your lover with abusive words? Yogis spend lifetimes contemplating *ahimsa*. I'm not sure if a life of nonviolence is possible, but considering our actions and being sensitive to their results is a start.

Those first couple of years in Bluffton tested practically every ethical precept in any system, whether it was the Christian commandment to "Love thy neighbor as thyself" or yoga's *yama* of nonviolence. Kids regularly threw eggs at our house. One day we woke up to find our car tires slashed and a piece of paper stuck to the windshield scrawled with the words: "When tires go flat, dago wop wop wop." (I had never heard the words *dago* or *wop*, but Mark explained them to me.) Later I heard that another sign had been posted on the bridge coming into Bluffton: "Blacks out of town BY SUNDOWN." Although I hate violence of any kind, I agree with *Bhagavad Gita*: there are times when not standing up to aggression is its own form of passive violence.

✦　✦　✦

Uprooting is a part of life. Stripping off our security blankets can create opportunities to experience the fresh air of the now. Most of us cling to what's familiar, which can stifle the possibility of spiritual growth. Trying to make something permanent often creates frustration and sadness because it's not possible. What we hold on to as fixed is in reality always changing—like trees through the seasons. The move to Bluffton jolted us out of our comfortable life in the way a meditation teacher might rap you with a stick to shock you out of daydreaming.

Fortunately, Mom and Dad created a stable home built on love. They adored each other; to this day, Dad tells the story about the first time he spotted my mom across the room at a school dance. She was a pretty sixteen-year-old Irish girl named Margaret Regina Kelly; her family and friends called her Jean. He was nineteen, had completed two years in the navy, and was finishing high school. He fell in love with her on the spot but was upset to learn she was so young. He wrote her a note, which he gave to her with a nickel and a bag of rocks. The note said that the nickel was for her to use to call him when she turned eighteen; the bag of rocks were to throw at any guy who tried to pick her up in the meantime. A year later, she sent a friend into a bar to ask my dad to come outside.

"Nick, I'm out of rocks," she said.

They went on their first date the next day.

A few months later, Dad was preparing to go to college on the GI Bill. Mom went to say good-bye to him. His car was packed, and he would be on his way in an hour.

"Will you wait for me?" he asked her.

"I'll be happy to see you when you're home, but I'm not making any promises. I'm going to date other guys," she said.

It was a no-brainer for Dad. He wasn't going to run the risk of losing his Irish honey. He unpacked the car and stayed, giving up the opportunity of a college education. He married Jean within the year.

I grew up thinking that all parents were as madly in love as mine. Even though Dad's work schedule was difficult, and they struggled with money issues, they had a deep and passionate relationship. He used to come up behind my mom at the dinner table, bend down, and whisper things in her ear that would make her giggle and blush. She'd pretend to swat him away. Dad used to joke, "Your mother gets pregnant every time I hang my pants on the bedpost!" For a while, my older sister, Peggy, thought that this was how babies were made.

Before long, the Zellos were legendary—an Italian Irish family with seven intelligent hippie kids in the middle of a conservative Indiana town. Teenage life in Bluffton was like a James Dean movie, with boys cruising up and down Main Street in their cars, revving their engines, and looking for girls. Our lives were filled with dates, basketball and baseball games, track-and-field events, church, and the school marching band (in which I played the drums).

Mom's children were her be-all and end-all. She was tiny but fierce, especially when she thought someone was messing with her tribe. My brothers all had long hair, and the police in Bluffton would grab boys like them and take them to the station house, where they'd give them buzz cuts. My parents almost never left town, but when my mom's father died and they were making plans to go to New York for the funeral, Mom marched into the police station and announced: "My sons have long hair today, and they damn well better have long hair when I get back." And they did.

In Bluffton, I could feel my mom's sadness despite her best efforts to conceal it. I started to internalize the feelings and focus on what I could control. I became a perfectionist, obsessed with getting good grades—both to please my parents and to be noticed in a house full of boys. By third grade, I was getting all A plusses; by the time I was eleven, I started experiencing stomach pains that were so intense they would make me double over. I was diagnosed with an ulcer.

One night when I was in junior high, my mother found me awake in my room at two in the morning, obsessively crumpling sheets of paper and rewriting my homework assignment over and over. "Colleen, there's nothing better than an A plus," she pleaded. "You have to go to sleep!" A few days later I came home with the assignment marked with an A++. From then on, my parents tried to bribe me to get Bs instead of As. It didn't work.

I sensed Mom had other heartaches as well, dark feelings that lurked in the recesses of her soul. Her family had been dirt poor and her father an alcoholic. She spent much of her childhood hungry, cold, and scared. She never talked to us about it. But when her brothers would visit, I would eavesdrop and listen to them telling stories about their father coming home drunk, and how he would yell and threateningly take off his belt and chase them around the house with it. I heard about the charities that would drop off clothes at their house, and Mom being ashamed to wear them—she weighed only eighty pounds at the time, so everything was huge on her. They recalled days when each child had only one slice of bread, and how my mother would flatten it to make it last longer, and put it under her pillow, taking one little piece at a time. They talked about Grandma breaking apart the kitchen table and burning it for heat when she thought her babies might freeze to death.

Near the end of my mom's life, I asked her if she would tell me about her childhood. She cried and said that when she would hear her father come home drunk late at night, she would hold her breath and pray that he wouldn't drag her out of her bed and force her to play the piano for him and his drunk buddies. Some of the puzzle was starting to make sense. Mom was a beautiful pianist, although the sound of her playing was haunting because she only played when she was sad. I know that her spiritual practice was strong, but her secrets and wounds and shame were buried deep in her body. Mr. Iyengar said that each of our bodies is a road map onto which all of our experiences are engraved. I believe that my mom's shame and heartbreak about her family history literally made her ill; she had heart disease, thyroid disease, varicose veins, colitis, and diverticulitis. Her religion didn't heal her sorrow—or her body.

I wish I could have wrung some of that trauma out of her body with an asana practice. A seated twist would have massaged her organs and brought fresh blood to them. A restorative backbend over a yoga bolster could have relieved her aching heart and opened her closed throat. Forward bends might have eased her stress and her blood pressure; backbends might have relieved her depression. In her last years, she was beginning to understand that yoga wasn't the devil's work or a cult. She even practiced chair yoga with a DVD I sent her. I love to think about my mom as a yogi.

Yoga Sequence: Grounding, Opening, Nurturing

When I designed this sequence, I went into our yoga room at home and put a photograph of Mom on the Tibetan chest Rodney and I use as an altar, alongside photos of our spiritual teachers: Mother Teresa, Swami Satchidananda, Mr. Iyengar, his brother-in-law Krishnamacharya, Pattabhi Jois, and Pema Chödrön. Alongside the pictures are my mother's and grandmother's rosaries, and a rosary blessed by Mother Teresa. I gaze at Mom's picture as I begin to imagine a sequence to ground us and respond to life's themes of rooting and uprooting, permanence and impermanence, attachment and separation. Foundation poses in yoga are important because they're the poses we keep coming back to, as to a mother. We move away from them and come back, move away and come back. We connect to the earth in these poses; when we stand in Mountain Pose, we feel the sensitivities of our own body. Which way does it sway? Where do we lose our balance? A mountain is strong, anchored, and inspiring. We look for these qualities as a foundation for our practice.

Tree Pose gives a sense of rooting and balancing while gazing. Even though my mother was uprooted geographically and emotionally, she still had strong roots in faith and her family. I've probably done Tree Pose ten thousand times, and I've felt my mom in every one.

Foundation poses inform our legs and our bodies to center us. Any time you feel off kilter is a time to do a foundation pose. If I've missed a flight, or if a business meeting has gone badly and I'm frustrated, I just stop and do Mountain Pose. I feel my feet. I watch my breath. It's the connection no one can take away from me. One of the challenges of yoga poses is to find the rooting, the body's central channel, from which flows steadiness, focus, and joy. Yet even as we find our grounding, we know we're part of nature, and that one of the few things we can be sure of is that everything is always changing.

This is also a sequence for anyone who feels depleted, or simply needs nurturing. You'll find yourself connecting to the ground while wringing out tension in the body. The sequence helps you see new possibilities, while you face the world with courage and tranquility.

List of Props needed for the sequences: yoga mat, 2 blocks, strap, 3 blankets, bolster (rolled-up blankets can substitute), 10-pound sandbag (or equal househould weight), chair.

Constructive Rest. Lie down on your back with your feet parallel and spread hip distance apart, knees bent and touching each other. Place your hands on your belly and watch the rise and fall of 10 breaths. For people who may be tired, this pose will ease them into the sequence. We don't stay long in the pose, because women like my mom are always moving pretty fast, and slowing down frightens them. This first pose gives a hint of slowing down.

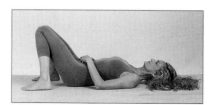

Constructive Rest

Stick Pose (yashtikasana). Raise your arms over your head and stretch your legs onto the floor. Reach your limbs in opposite directions until you feel a slight hollowing in your lower belly (between your pubis and navel). Continue for 5 breaths. It's important for our back bodies to be in contact with the ground in order to feel the support and connection to the supreme mother-earth. I imagine my mother feeling grounded and held in this pose.

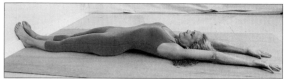

Stick Pose

Thunderbolt Pose (vajrasana). Kneel and sit back on your heels. Interlace your fingers and reach your arms overhead with the palms facing the ceiling for 3 breaths. Exhale the arms down, change the interlace so the other index finger is on top, and reach up again for 3 more breaths. This will initiate the pattern of folding the legs in preparation for Tree Pose later in the sequence.

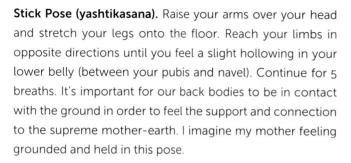

Thunderbolt Pose

Mountain Pose (tadasana). Stand with your feet firmly planted, arms hanging alongside the torso. Feel how your weight subtly shifts from side to side, front to back. Feel your roots grow deeper. From the foundation of your legs, float your torso up and balance your head above your spine. Inhale, feel your feet, exhale, and feel your chest. Stay for 10 breaths.

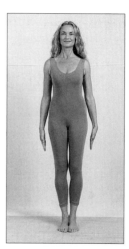

Mountain Pose

Volcano Pose (urdhva hastasana). In Mountain, inhale and reach your arms actively upward. This is the start of stretching up from our roots, trusting that we have a solid foundation from which to extend. Elongate from the waist and try to touch the ceiling with your fingertips. Inhale, feel how your feet contact the floor, exhale, and take your arms higher until you feel a hollow in your lower belly. Hold for 5 breaths.

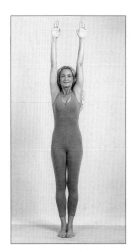

Volcano Pose

Tree Pose (vrikshasana). Spend another 3 breaths in Mountain, continue to feel your feet growing down like roots into the floor. Then bend your right knee and take your right foot to the inside of your left thigh, as high as is comfortable. Reach your arms straight up alongside your ears. Keep the feeling of floating your chest and head. Watch yourself grow down through your roots into the floor while balancing on one leg. Focus on something about 6 feet in front of you that isn't moving. My mom was a worrier, so the simplicity and challenge of balancing in this pose would have created an opportunity, in the words of Ram Dass, for her to "Be Here Now." Don't be rigid as you stay for 5 breaths. Lower the foot to the floor and repeat on the left side for 5 breaths.

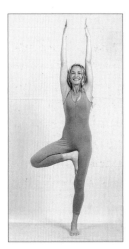

Tree Pose

Sit in **Staff Pose (dandasana),** both legs straight and active, torso upright (a). Then move into **Bent-Knee Seated Twist (marichyasana III)** by folding your left leg and standing the heel as close to the left sitting bone as possible (b). Twist easily to the left and hug your left knee with your right arm. Twists serve as a form of therapeutic massage for the body's organs of digestion and elimination. Hold for 5 breaths and repeat to the right. Then return to Staff.

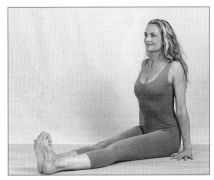

Staff Pose (a)

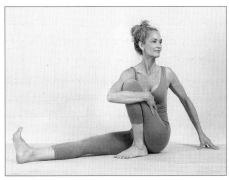

Bent-Knee Seated Twist (b)

Bound Angle Pose (baddha konasana). Sit down and place the soles of your feet together as you drop your knees open. Draw your heels as close to your pelvis as is comfortable. As you inhale, lift your knees up slightly and firmly press the inner heels. As you exhale, press your outer heels and let the knees release. This pose is good for digestion and my mom would have benefited from it. Stay for 10 cycles of breath.

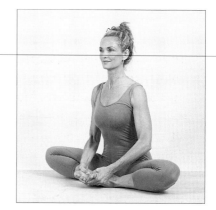

Bound Angle Pose

Supported Fish Pose (matsyasana). Place a rolled-up blanket or bolster horizontally across your mat and lie over it with the bolster under your shoulder blades. Rest your head on the floor; if your neck is uncomfortable, place your head on a folded blanket. Take your arms out to the sides with your elbows bent and your palms facing up. When people are depressed, inhalation becomes shallow and difficult. This pose opens the chest and makes breathing easier; it's life-affirming. Enjoy for 15 breaths.

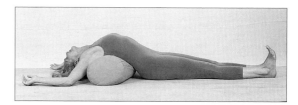

Supported Fish Pose

Legs Up the Wall (viparita karani mudra). Position a folded blanket about 3 inches from the wall and lie down with your sacrum on the blanket and your legs up the wall (a). Your sitting bones should hang in the space between the blanket and the wall, which will give your front torso a smooth arch from the pubis to the shoulders. If you have tight hamstrings, bend your knees a little or move farther from the wall (b). My mom's legs were riddled with painful varicose veins and her heart was taxed. An inverted pose helps with the venous return of the blood from the lower body, which would have eased the pressure in her legs and improved the blood flow back to her heart. The chest is lifted so that the breath is easy. Dropping the head below a lifted chest has a calming effect on the body. I have found this to be a miraculous pose in times of stress or fatigue. Hold for about 3 minutes.

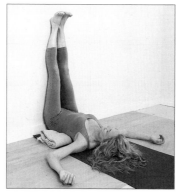

Legs Up Wall (a)

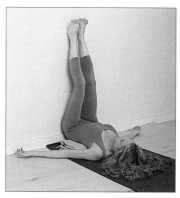

Legs Up Wall Variation (b)

Final Relaxation (shavasana). Lie on your back with your legs straight, heels slightly apart (a). Wiggle around until you're comfortable, then place your arms alongside your torso with your palms facing up. For optimal restoration, strap your thighs together with a belt, put sandbags or weights on them, and cover your eyes with a small pillow (b). Stay in the pose for 5 to 10 minutes, relaxing your body and letting go of all tension.

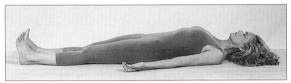

Final Relaxation (a)

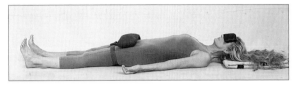

Final Relaxation Variation (b)

The goal of this sequence is to get us in touch with our inherent physical strength and balance, qualities that can ground us through the upheavals of life. I imagine it could have given my mother courage, support, and connectivity. Mom, you held so many of us; here is a sequence that will hold you and everyone who's in need of steadiness and joy.

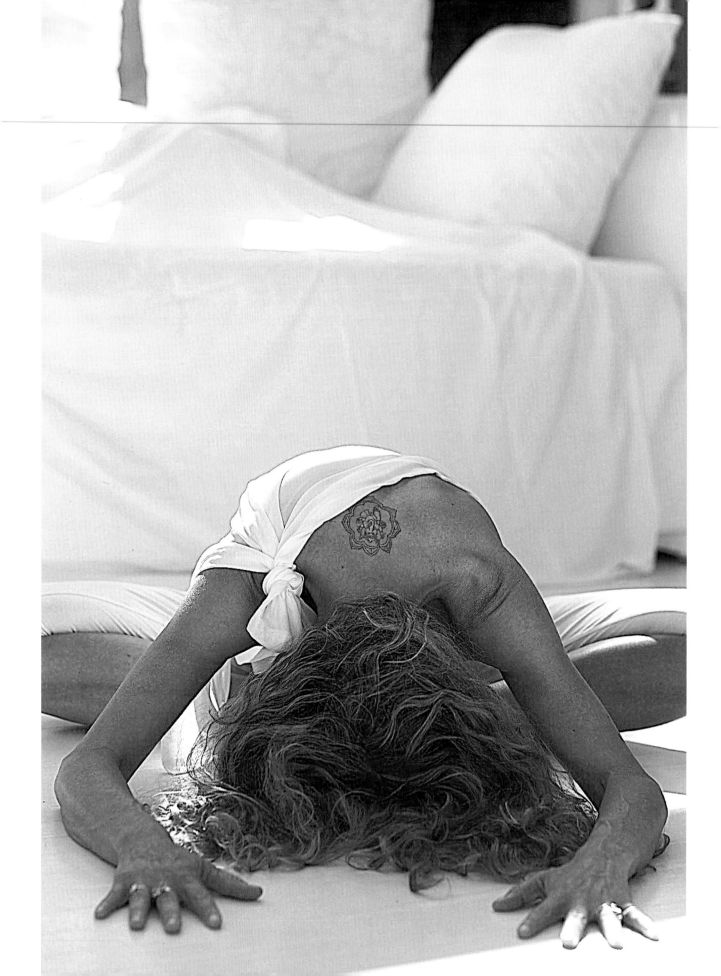

Chapter 2

TRAUMA

Silence is an empty space,
Space is the home of the awakened mind.

—Buddha

On the Fourth of July weekend when I was fifteen years old, I was with a group of friends chicken-racing down the middle of Highway 124 at dusk. A driver coming over the rise either didn't see us or couldn't stop fast enough and barreled into us. The impact sent bodies flying into the air in all directions. One of my girlfriends suffered a broken back, another a fractured pelvis, and I sustained a skull fracture and a broken collarbone. When I'd landed, I skidded across the pavement, scraping most of the skin off one side of my body.

My parents had gone to a party in Angola, Indiana, about an hour and a half from Bluffton. I had recently gotten into drugs, and that afternoon my friends and I had gone to the house of a local dealer. A beautiful brunette who looked like Pocahontas opened the door. We bought some acid called "Love" and some Quaaludes.

Pretty soon we were tripping and chicken-racing. Three teams with one person on the shoulders of another were running side by side, trying to knock each other off. Laughing and careening into one another, trying to be the last one standing, we never saw the car coming.

My older brother Joe was at a party with friends that evening. Someone at the party heard there had been an accident and that I might be involved. Joe rushed to the hospital and gave the doctors permission to do more than just stop the bleeding. Drifting in and out of consciousness in the ER, I became aware that the monsignor from our church had appeared beside me. According to people who were there, he asked about administering last rites, and I said, "I'm not going to die, Monsignor. So, please, get the hell out of here."

The only thing I remember about my stay in the hospital is screaming when the nurses changed my bandages—it was so painful. While the doctors and my family focused on my physical injuries, I was more scared about what was happening to my brain: I couldn't remember anything. I couldn't think clearly. The world seemed to be going along just as before, but inside I wasn't the same.

Shortly after I was released, I went to a party (which we called a "kegger"). My head was still partly shaved where my scalp had been sutured and I was wearing an orange-and-white-checkered halter top with a shoulder harness over it that held my broken collarbone. The whole right side of my body was covered with bandages. I felt like some girl Frankenstein.

A plastic cup of beer was in my hand and I was swaying to the music. I lived for music; like all my siblings I worshiped Bob Dylan and knew the lyrics to all his songs by heart. Now I couldn't even remember the first verse to "Blowin' in the Wind."

When I went back to school for my sophomore year in the fall, I had trouble concentrating. I'd been a straight-A+ student before the accident. Now, I had to study incredibly hard to get a B and sometimes even a C, which was as good as an F to me. I knew that, in some way, my brain was damaged.

Frustration in life is inescapable. We've all had the experience of losing something that we would desperately like to have back. The yearning creates internal anxiety, depression, low self-esteem, and conflict. I wasn't able to accept this new reality and the post-accident brain I now had. I was also suffering from post-traumatic stress disorder (PTSD), though no one diagnosed it at the time. For years afterward, the sound of screeching car brakes became a trigger for intense anxiety and panic. Sometimes, just lying in bed at night and hearing a car drive by would be enough to make me freeze and shake violently in terror.

I needed relief. After the accident, I found that one of the most therapeutic activities I could do was running. I'd been an accomplished runner since I was eight years old when I'd won a 50-yard dash at a Junior Olympics–type event in Watkins Glen, New York. Even after the accident, I set records at Bluffton High School in the 50-yard dash, 100-yard dash, anchor leg on the 440, as well as hurdles, long jump, and high jump. Some of those records stood for thirty years.

Running had always put me into a kind of trance. It was one of my first meditative experiences, and it let me escape from my self-berating, never-good-enough routine. Running produces endorphins that are calming; running lowers anxiety. I loved the feeling I had when I ran. It was shelter from the storm.

Running also made me feel seen. Because I had so many siblings, excelling at something was a way to stand out. Later, the sweet and intense rush of drugs hitting my veins would remind me of the feeling of running, of breaking the tape at a finish line—the world slows down and becomes beautiful.

I also found relief in prayer. Good Catholics that we were, our family went to confession every Saturday, Mass every Sunday, and we kids attended catechism classes on Wednesday evenings. My brothers couldn't have cared less about praying but went through the motions to please my mom. I loved praying. I shared a bedroom with my older sister Peggy, and being younger, had to go to bed earlier than she did. I'd pull the blankets over my head and repeat, over and over, "Hail Mary, full of grace. The Lord is with thee. Blessed art thou amongst women, and blessed is the fruit of thy womb, Jesus. Holy Mary, Mother of God, pray for us sinners, now and at the hour of our death." The Hail Mary was my first mantra. I thought if I could just pray enough, everything would turn out okay: Bluffton, Dad's job, Mom's tears—and me.

Soon, drugs gave me more relief than either running or prayer. I started with marijuana and quickly moved on to hashish and alcohol. Before long, I was dabbling in hallucinogens (mescaline and acid). With drugs, people tend to gravitate to one end of the energetic spectrum or the other. Some prefer uppers—like speed and cocaine—and others like downers, such as Quaaludes, which became my drug of choice. They made me feel comfortable, relaxed, and sexy.

We can choose among many paths in life. Each of us is looking for one that feels right, that fits our sensibilities, that will help alleviate our suffering, and maybe even create a little enlightenment. My mother had the Catholic Church with its rituals and Ten Commandments. My friends who are Buddhists follow the Eightfold Path with its meditation, right speech, right intention, and right action. Yogis have *ashtanga*, the "eight limbs" for how to live a meaningful and purposeful life.

✦   ✦   ✦

If my accident at age fifteen had any upside, it's that I have a heightened empathy for the traumas, large and small, that my students have experienced. At times, I can see where trauma is held in their bodies, and I try to figure out sequences that can create relief and release for them. Trauma can show up as tension, anxiety, or illness. Some common places of binding are the pelvis, the diaphragm, the throat, the jaw, the hamstrings, and the shoulders and neck. I can sense trauma in a student's choppy breath or darting eyes. When we release the "stuck" areas in our bodies, we're better able to glimpse what yoga calls the true or authentic self. This is a big part of why we step onto the mat: we're looking for freedom from the imprints and obstructions that are held in our bodies. We intuit that we're not free, but we don't know why.

When we practice yoga, we learn that we can sit with our traumas and observe them instead of trying to run from them. We notice where the blockages and obstacles in our bodies are, and we recognize the stories we create to hold them there. Physical injuries can create scar tissue. Fear and grief and pain also can create debilitating, invisible scar tissue. Yoga practice often brings these unconscious blockages to the surface and helps release them.

In order to unlock these areas of tension slowly, methodically, and mindfully, it's important to sequence yoga poses correctly. With care, we can chip away at habitual ways of being in the world that cause us isolation and suffering. Yoga sequences are designed to uncover our birthright: love, joy, and freedom. The body can experience these essences as space, ease, and liberation.

For many people, yoga is simply stretching or exercising. It is that, but it's also so much more. Why do we put our bodies in strange poses that are uncomfortable and challenging? Why do we practice meditation, which can be even more difficult than the physical practice of yoga? Asana wrings stress and tension out of the body—then we sit in meditation with what arises. We attempt to observe ourselves calmly without running, knowing that the fear of the imaginary is often much worse than the reality. As Mark Twain put it, "I am an old man and have known a great many troubles, but most of them never happened."

Like the Department of Homeland Security, our bodies have their own voluminous manuals of "just in case" defenses. Armor builds up around pain and makes us hard, alienated, and sick. The mind is brilliant at making up stories that explain and justify our armor—and these can paralyze us. Our stories are what Patanjali, who compiled the *Yoga Sutras*, calls the *citta vritti*, the "fluctuations of the mind."

The first step toward liberation is to realize that we have this incessant "monkey mind," or chatter, going on in our heads. Instead of becoming prisoner to it, we can use yoga to help us develop the ability to witness our habits and our habitual responses. When we practice the eight limbs of yoga, our minds quiet, like a child who's being held. As the surface ripples on the lake calm, we see the jewel that sits obscured in our hearts. This is what we do on our yoga mats: we sit with what is here and now so that we can become vulnerable, exposed, and real. As the stories buried in our bodies emerge, we open up space for them so they don't have the same hold over us. With that perspective, we can see our own beauty. As the Persian poet Hafiz writes: "There are so many unopened gifts from our birthday." Do we want to die with our gifts—our potential—locked inside us?

The first thing to notice is where the dumping grounds in your body are; there can be many, and they change. My dumping ground as a child was my belly—and I got an ulcer in the third grade. Later, my dumping ground became my throat—I was scared to talk for fear of looking stupid. After that, it was my back—I didn't feel supported. And now it's my shoulders—I carry the weight of motherhood, marriage, and a business.

During my Jivamukti Yoga Teacher Training, I had the privilege of meeting Sri Swami Satchidananda, a renowned Indian spiritual teacher who developed a system he called Integral Yoga. Satchidananda said that when we are practicing *pranayama* (a channeling of the *prana* or "life force" through breath work), we are closest to God during the pause at the end of the exhalation. He explained that the pause *is* the experience of space and peace.

Yoga is about the search for space, physically and emotionally. We aren't trying to erase our stories, but to place them in a larger context. What happens when you put a teaspoon of salt into a cup of water? The water becomes highly salty. What happens when you put a teaspoon of salt into a lake? The teaspoon of salt is still there, but its impact is minimal.

In yoga, we aim to become the lake, to put our problems and issues into that larger context so we aren't thrown off balance as easily, so we can keep connected to our centers. Looking to expand our perspective on personal suffering, the Vietnamese Zen monk Thich Nhat Hanh once said, "Even as they kill my people, a flower blooms." My mom used to say that her heart grew bigger with every baby—that there was plenty of love for us all.

After my accident on Highway 124, my brain never worked the same way again. I became a different person as a result, but I now understand that I'm more than just the part of my brain that was damaged. My dance today is complete, fulfilling, and maybe even more interesting and beautiful as a result. There are days when I can barely taste the salt because my lake is big enough. "Enlightenment feels like spaciousness in the joints," Swami Satchidananda said. How lovely when we begin to feel it.

Yoga Sequence: Relief from Anxiety and Trauma

During a workshop several years ago, Rodney picked up a small wooden mallet that goes with the singing bowl we keep at the studio and began lightly tapping his hand with it to engender steady breath. A student came up to him during the break and asked him to please stop. Fifteen minutes later, I noticed that she had left the class. I went outside to look for her and found her on the ground, curled up in a fetal position, crying. Later we found out that her boyfriend had beaten her with a bat; the mallet Rodney was holding had triggered her post-traumatic stress.

At first I could tell she didn't want to be disturbed. I left her where she was and grabbed several yoga blankets and wrapped her in them. I instructed her to keep her eyes open and asked her if she knew where she was and to tell me the color of the car that was parked nearby. When someone is having a traumatic flashback or suffering an anxiety attack, it's important for the person to keep his or her eyes open; otherwise the traumatic scene can replay itself. As she became more responsive, the immediate trauma began to subside.

In this relief sequence, we generally ask people to keep their backs to the wall and their eyes open to promote a feeling of safety; they can see the room in front of them and are reassured that they are not in present danger. Body scan meditation is a helpful technique in which you notice different parts of your body and related sensations that are occurring. You can start a body scan with these questions: Do I feel my feet? Are they warm or cold?

Anxiety and PTSD create tension in the back, neck, and shoulders, as well as tightness in the hips and hamstrings. There are days when the body is flooded with the stress hormones cortisol and epinephrine; activities such as meditation or yoga are known to reduce stress and can help us quiet anxiety and trauma one breath and one posture at a time. Even practicing something as simple as pausing after your exhalation for ten minutes a day can add up to a substantial period of relief from grief, fear, or anxiety. It also can empower you to realize there's something you can do to help yourself. None of us is powerless.

Mountain Pose (tadasana). Stand with your back to the wall in Mountain for 2 regular breaths (a). Exhale and hug your right knee into your belly (b). Set the foot down as you inhale, and with an exhale, hug your left knee into your belly. Inhale and set your left foot down. Repeat 4 times on each side. This will move you strongly into your legs and the folding will prepare you for Tree Pose (vrikshasana).

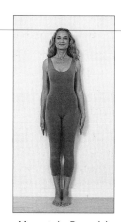 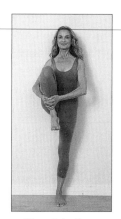 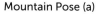

Mountain Pose (a)

Mountain Pose Variation (b)

Tree Pose (vrikshasana). Continue standing with the back of your torso against the wall. Hug your right knee into your belly and then place your right foot as high up your left inner thigh as possible. Press your palms together in front of your chest in prayer position—this helps you avoid feeling exposed and vulnerable. Stay for 5 breaths and repeat with the left leg. Because balance is challenging in Tree Pose, it demands your attention, which fixes your mind in the present.

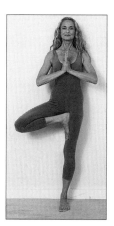

Tree Pose

Chair Pose with Eagle Arms (utkatasana with garudasana arms). With your back still against a wall, walk your feet 6 inches out and bend your knees as if beginning to sit down onto a chair. Bend your elbows and bring the left elbow into the crook of the right, backs of your hands facing each other. Then pass your left hand in front of your right and bring the palms together, thumbs pointing toward the tip of your nose. (Grab your wrist if you can't press your palms together.) Hold for 5 breaths, then reverse your arms and hold for 5 breaths. This is a challenging pose that keeps the mind attentive and requires strong use of the legs. The arms in Eagle release tension in the upper back muscles between the shoulder blades. The wall behind you and your arms in front of you create a feeling of safety. As you inhale, lift your elbows slightly. As you exhale, bend your knees a little more deeply.

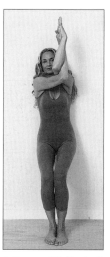

Chair Pose with Eagle Arms

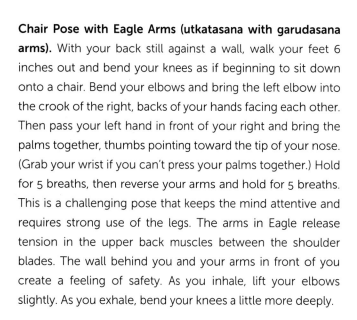

Modified Sun Salutation (surya namaskar). In this trauma sequence we don't reach the arms overhead because that can leave the body feeling vulnerable. Stand at the front of your mat in **Mountain Pose** (a). Fold forward **Modified Standing Forward Bend** (b) by placing your hands on a block, knees slightly bent. Bend your knees more as you look forward. Step your right foot back to a **Lunge** (c), then move into **Downward-Facing Dog** (d) for 5 breaths. Step the right foot forward, then your left, and return to **Standing Forward Bend** (e). Continue to use the modified version if you feel any strain in your lower back. Put your hands on your hips and use your legs to come to stand in **Mountain Pose** (f). To repeat on the other side, step your left foot back into a lunge, and finish in Mountain Pose. Sun Salutation is a simple way to link breath with movement and release tension while keeping your mind focused. It also improves circulation and burns up nervous energy.

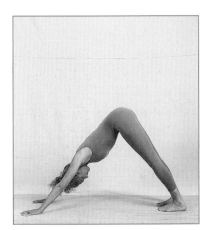

Mountain Pose (a)

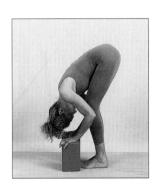

Modified Standing
Forward Bend (b)

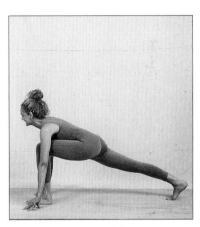

Lunge (c)

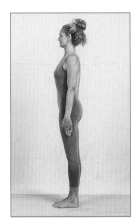

Downward-Facing Dog (d)

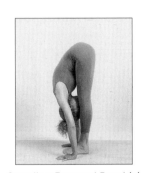

Standing Forward Bend (e)

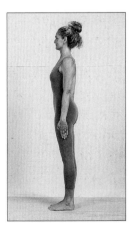

Mountain Pose (f)

Warrior II (virabhadrasana II). Step your right foot forward, then pivot on the ball of the left foot and press your left heel firmly on the floor and into the wall. Spiral your arms up parallel to the floor as your hips open to the side. Bend your front knee to a 90-degree angle. Hold for 5 breaths, then lower your hands to either side of your front foot and step back to Downward-Facing Dog. Repeat on the left side, then walk forward to Standing Forward Bend.

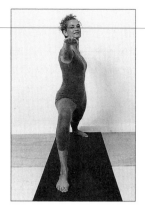

Warrior II

Modified Warrior I (virabhadrasana I). From Standing Forward Bend, step your left foot back, then your right into Downward-Facing Dog. Step your right foot forward between your hands, knee as close to 90 degrees as possible, and press your left heel to the floor and the wall. Lift your torso to upright, but keep your hips facing the front of the mat. Take your hands to prayer position in front of your chest (again, we keep the arms low in order to promote a feeling of safety). Hold for 5 breaths, then take your hands to the floor and step back to Downward-Facing Dog. Repeat on the other side, hold again for 5 breaths, return to Downward-Facing Dog, and walk forward to Standing Forward Bend.

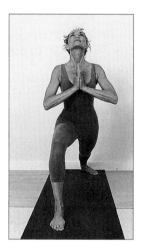

Modified Warrior I

Warrior III (virabhadrasana III). From Standing Forward Bend, step back into Downward-Facing Dog. Step your right foot forward and lift into Warrior I with your hands on your hips. Lay your torso on your right thigh, and with an inhale, reach your arms forward, straighten your right leg and lift the left leg parallel to the floor, pressing your left foot strongly into the wall for Warrior III. Look forward and reach strongly through your lifted leg. Hold for 3 breaths, step down to Warrior I, then to Downward-Facing Dog. Repeat on the other side, and walk forward to Standing Forward Bend. These three Warrior poses strengthen the legs and help focus the mind in the present.

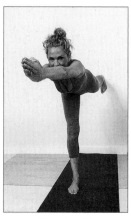

Warrior III

Modified Raised Leg Stretch Pose (utthita hasta padangushthasana) with a chair. With your back to the wall, stand facing the chair. Inhale, lift your right foot, and rest it on the seat. Then lean forward and rest your hands on the back of the chair. Hold for 10 breaths and repeat on the other side. This forward bend calms your nervous system and starts the process of releasing your hamstrings, our fight-or-flight responders. Looking into the room keeps your mind in the here and now and the chair offers a protective barrier.

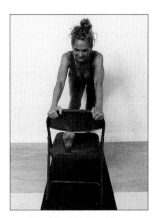

Modified Raised Leg
Stretch Pose

Wide-Legged Seated Forward Bend (upavishtha konasana) with a chair. With your back against the wall, open your legs to a wide straddle. Position a chair in front of you between your legs, then rest your crossed forearms on a blanket on the front edge of the seat and rest your chin on the arms in Wide-Legged Seated Forward Bend (a). Keep your mind focused by gazing at something in front of you. Then rest your forehead on the chair and drape your arms over the chair's seat to relax the neck in a variation of the pose (b). This releases the inner thigh muscles and hamstrings, which are two of the muscle groups that fire when we feel stress or panic. Stay for 20 breaths.

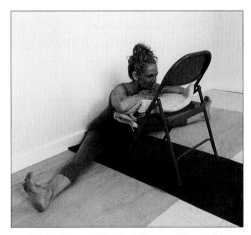

Wide-Legged Seated Forward Bend (a)

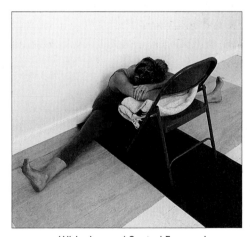

Wide-Legged Seated Forward
Bend Variation (b)

Bent-Knee Seated Forward Bend (janu shirshasana) with a chair. Sit on a folded blanket, bend your right knee deeply, and lay your outer leg on the floor, your shin at approximately a right angle to your straight left leg. Place the chair over your straight leg and fold forward, resting your forehead on the chair (a). If the bare seat is uncomfortable, pad it with a towel or blanket. You can rest your forehead on the chair and gaze at the floor, or rest your chin on the chair and look into the room in a variation of the pose (b). Drape your arms over the chair. This pose continues the work of releasing the hamstrings and inner thighs. Stay for 15 breaths on each side.

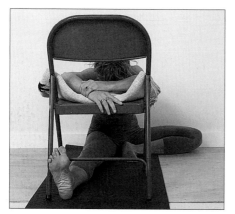

Bent-Knee Seated Forward Bend (a)

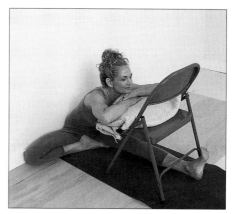

Bent-Knee Seated Forward Bend Variation (b)

Easy Pose (sukhasana) with a chair. Sit on the edge of a folded blanket, your right shin crossed in front of your left, and fold forward, resting your head and arms on a chair, eyes open. As much as possible, relax your hips and back muscles. This pose releases tension, quiets the nervous system, and initiates the process of turning inward. Notice your breath, how your back lifts as you inhale and drops as you exhale. Stay for 10 breaths and repeat with your left shin in front of your right.

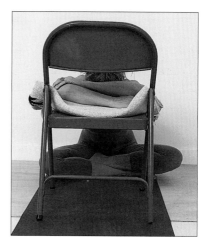

Easy Pose with a Forward Bend

Child's Pose (balasana). Sit on your heels facing away from the wall and spread your knees wider than shoulder distance apart. Pull the end of a bolster into your inner thighs and lie over it. Turn your head to one side and keep your eyes open. This pose encourages full exhalation, which helps alleviate anxiety. Do a simple body scan meditation by naming the parts of your body, either aloud or silently. Count the length of your exhalation. Stay for 2 minutes, then turn your head to the opposite side and stay for 2 more minutes.

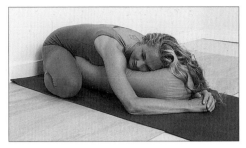

Child's Pose

Final Relaxation (shavasana) with chair. Lie down on your back and rest your calves on the seat of the chair. Cross your arms in front of your torso as if hugging yourself. We release the calves (another fight-or-flight muscle) during this version of the pose, which enables us to drop deeper into our inner journey. Keep your eyes open and focus softly on something above you. Observe the sensations that come over you and watch them pass like clouds. Notice that the present moment isn't full of demons. Scan the body from the head to the feet. If you're agitated, return to a cross-legged seated position. Stay for 5 minutes in either pose.

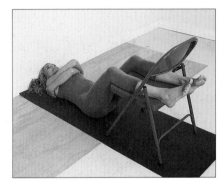

Final Relaxation

Meditation (dhyana). Sit cross-legged on a folded blanket or with your back against the wall and your eyes open. Focus on your breath and body and softly observe the natural pause at the end of the exhalation while gazing at something in the room. Stay for 2 minutes.

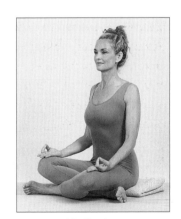

Meditation

For everyone who may be suffering physical or emotional trauma, this sequence can help create relief with the benefits of focus, relaxation, and a feeling of safety.

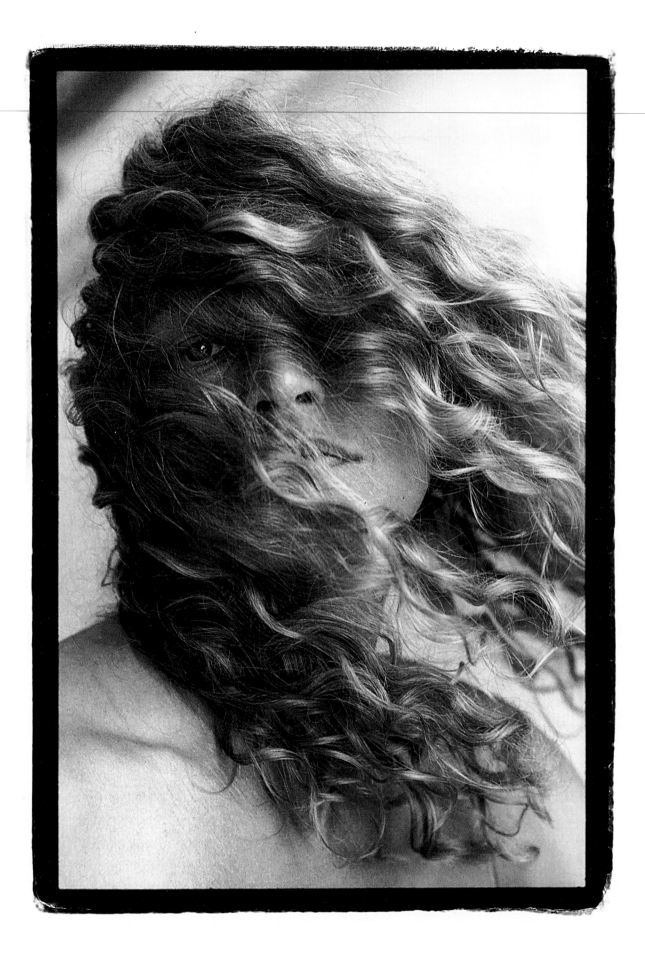

Chapter 3

ADDICTION

There is no coming to consciousness without pain.
People will do anything, no matter how absurd, to avoid facing their own soul.
One does not become enlightened by imagining figures of light,
but by making the darkness conscious.

—Carl Jung

There were several of us passed out on a huge octagon-shaped waterbed, nearing the end of a three-day heroin blackout, when Dad called. I answered the phone in a stupor and he told me in no uncertain terms that he expected to see me at my brother Nick's high school graduation later that afternoon.

The year before, 1978, I'd dropped out of my freshman year at Ball State University in Muncie, Indiana, and married my boyfriend, a drummer in a rock band. Jeff had beautiful eyes and drove a fancy car with shiny mag wheels and loud woofers. He was the coolest guy, and I was totally smitten.

I had been miserable during my nine months at college. I would leave every Friday to go home and I'd get hives every Sunday evening when I had to go back. I wanted to spend all of my time with Jeff and the band. Drugs were big in my repertoire of activities. Everywhere I went it seemed there was a coffee table with a mirror, rolled-up dollar bills, and lines of cocaine. It wasn't long before heroin made its way into the mix. I partied like crazy. One of the girls who used to hang out with the band was a heavy user—the kind who sometimes didn't even bother to take the strap off her arm between fixes. I adored her. We were like sisters. One day I went to visit her on my lunch break and found her freaking out because she couldn't find a vein undamaged enough to take the syringe. She asked me to do her a favor and shoot her up in her eye. I was shocked, but I managed to do it because I wanted to help her. I'm still amazed at the intensity of her need and how far she was willing to go to get relief.

On my father's order, I showed up at Nick's graduation. Unfortunately, I was wearing a thin, white polyester jumpsuit inside out, unbuttoned to my navel with no underwear. I was high as a kite and staggering around, occasionally using the wall to brace myself. Mom thought I was drunk and asked Peggy to make sure that I didn't come to the graduation party at our house. Peggy told Mom and Dad that she was terrified I was in over my head with drugs. When she let me know that I wasn't to attend the party, she admitted she had told our parents I was drugged-out. A few days later Dad called and said he wanted me in rehab. I thought that was insane and told Jeff that we had to get out of town.

I felt betrayed by Peggy. We had always had each other's backs. Why would she squeal on me? The poet Hafiz wrote: "Dear One, wise up. Blame keeps the sad game going." It would take me a while to see that she probably saved my life.

Jeff and I had always talked about living in New York City, so we packed a couple of suitcases, got in the car, and started driving. The biggest city either of us had been to up to that point was Fort Wayne, Indiana. So, like the Clampetts driving into Los Angeles in their old jalopy in the opening scene of *The Beverly Hillbillies*, Jeff and I headed to Manhattan, except we were about as far from newly minted millionaires as you could get. "Wow," I said, as we approached Times Square. "This is where the ball drops!"

In the Zello family, New Year's Eve was always a big deal. Mom and Dad would come home from a party to be with us kids at midnight. Dad would film the ball dropping on the TV screen and pan the video camera around the room of sleepy children. As the clock struck midnight, Mom and Dad would kiss for way too long, and we would squeal and throw our party favors at them. To be in New York City in real life was mind-blowing.

Times Square then wasn't the glittering tourist mecca it is today, but was gritty and dangerous. Jeff and I checked into a rundown hotel called the Piccadilly on West Forty-Fifth Street. We had no plans. We dragged our suitcases to the room and I settled down to get high. Bryant Park, a drug haven at the time, was just a few blocks away.

Just a year before I'd sat with my father on the porch of our house in Bluffton and told him I was going to quit college and marry Jeff. "Colleen," he said, with his head in his hands. "You're still a teenager. I'll give you everything I have in my bank account—three thousand dollars—if you don't do this. Please, listen to me." I tuned him out as he tried to change my mind. Then he started to cry. It was the first time I'd ever seen my dad break down. His face crumpled in anguish as I insisted on going through with the marriage. The agony I caused him haunts me to this day.

The morning after Jeff and I arrived at the Piccadilly, I woke up jumpy and agitated, a sensation that was becoming all too familiar. I had gotten to a place where I needed drugs to feel like myself. My mind started to race. I had a little money from a job I'd had in Indiana selling advertising for a newspaper called *Farmers' Advance.* Jeff had some cash from a regular gig he'd had, but even together, we didn't have enough money to sustain life in a hotel, much less in New York City. The money we spent in one day in Manhattan could have supported us for a month back home. What were we going to do? I didn't have any real skills. Suddenly something occurred to me. I knew a few girls in Indiana who were making good money working at strip clubs, with big tips from what they called "add-ons" in the back room. I was one fix and one blow job away from heading down that path.

It still shocks me that the idea of selling sex even entered my mind. *Who had I become?* Yet thirty-five years later, I can laugh at the thought that, even in the desperation of that moment, I was thinking in business terms. Thank God, I didn't act on it. I've always been practical. I had never wanted to live like my parents, sitting in the kitchen with the checkbook, bills strewn over the table, agonizing over which ones they could afford to pay at the end of the month. When I was ten years old, I decided to help them by babysitting and mowing lawns. When I was fourteen, I got a job at Coopers' Rest Home as an assistant activities director. I loved being with older people and felt that I was making a contribution by doing rounds and entertaining them with funny faces with sequins on Styrofoam balls.

That day, something clicked. I walked down the hallway to the shared bathroom, locked the door, looked in the mirror, and started to cry. I was Colleen Zello, a Midwestern Catholic high school track star with two parents who adored her and a sister and five brothers who would have killed for her. I didn't recognize the girl staring back at me. I didn't want to get high anymore, but I didn't know what to do. So I took a bath.

I don't know how long I stayed in there, only that I felt safe. Over the next several days, I quit heroin cold turkey. Other guests knocked on the bathroom door and yelled things like, "What's going on?" or "When are you coming out?!" I itched. I vomited. I shook. I felt as if I had something physical in my body that I had to expel.

The worst part of that time wasn't kicking heroin; it was the memory of the look in my father's eyes seeing me at Nick's graduation—his desperation, his agony. Knowing I had caused him that kind of pain shocked me enough to pull my head out of my ass. This man had sacrificed everything for us. I couldn't inflict more misery on him, or on the rest of my family. I didn't want to become alienated from the people I loved most. I had to stop doing drugs and reckon with myself.

◆   ◆   ◆

The Buddhist nun Pema Chödrön talks about the need for people to face the damage that their actions cause. Carl Jung wrote that until we come face-to-face with our "shadow"—the dark side of our nature that's hidden from our consciousness and driven by primitive urges such as anger, rage, lust, selfishness—there can be no transformation. If enlightenment means that the ego has been flattened, I was there. I had hit bottom. Many teachings say that the greatest opportunity lies there. I'm not sure I could have sunk any lower and been able to dig myself out.

This may be the strongest yoga lesson of all: the realization that selfishness and self-destruction affect everyone around you. Waking up to the fact that I was hurting others gave me a kick in the pants and the resolve to stop.

Today, many people who are struggling with addiction come to Rodney's and my classes—whether their addiction is to food, relationships, sex, power, alcohol, or drugs. Addiction seems to be part of the human condition. Our good friend Dr. Robby Stein, a psychologist, says we all are looking for things that will bring us relief from pain. Whatever we choose creates a particular feeling—a neurologic pathway that Robby calls a "river in the sand." We associate the substance with decreased anxiety, relief, and pleasure. Whatever our drug of choice, we repeat the behavior, which cuts deeper and deeper gorges into our psyches until the dependence becomes rigidly fixed. We become prisoners of our habits. The actions we take to alleviate our suffering create imprints called *samskaras*—the yogic version of Robby's "rivers." We have a beer, a joint, a cigarette, a Snickers bar, and we feel better. So we have another. Behavior becomes habit, but the relief is always temporary; it never solves the original problem, which is our pain and alienation from ourselves.

The most successful recovery programs are based on helping the addicted person uncover a spiritual dimension. We can call that dimension by any number of names—a higher power, God, the divine. In yoga, we see the true self as transcendent. The work we do to uncover that part of us holds the promise of transformation, liberation, and maybe even enlightenment. The eighth and ultimate limb of yoga, *samadhi*, is complete absorption in that state—no separation.

◆　　◆　　◆

For a long time, drugs were my habit and my relief. I did some kind of drug every day for four years. The first time heroin entered my bloodstream, I thought, *This is the end of my suffering.* Quaaludes made me feel comfortable and sexy in my body, but heroin was something entirely different. Someone accurately described its effect as "being wrapped in God's warmest blanket."

Addiction is a form of running away from feeling. What are the sensations we need to escape? What substances do we use to numb ourselves? Is the pain of life that unbearable? Have we become so disconnected from ourselves and from each other that we feel hopelessly alienated and lonely? I was looking for a way out of the intensity of feelings, whether they were confusion about my mom's sadness, or frustration over my brain, or shame about quitting college. In yoga and meditation, we learn to sit with our feelings. We notice where the sensation is and how it changes. We let go of the story that goes with the sensation. To know that a feeling will likely pass, no matter how irritating or painful it is, without needing to find relief from it, is liberation. That is tuning *in*, rather than tuning *out*.

In one of the first yoga workshops I took with Rodney, he said, "We all have a place inside of us that's unbearable to touch. So we lock it away. Through our yoga practice, we start to touch that place. Slowly, we open the hidden compartments of shame, grief, and trauma that are buried in our bodies."

There's a reason contemplative traditions eschew artificially altered states of consciousness. The bliss of asana, *pranayama*, and meditation supplant any chemical high.

Today I joke that I get my kicks by staying up late and watching Iyengar yoga videos. Mr. Iyengar, who died last year at ninety-five, was a savant about the body. In one video, an interviewer follows him around asking questions, and you can see him becoming annoyed. The interviewer asks, "Mr. Iyengar, why isn't the kind of yoga you teach spiritual?" He gives him a long stare and replies, "Have you ever been aware of every cell in your body equally? No? Well, once you have, please come back and tell me if that experience isn't spiritual."

Several summers ago, I was invited to help lead an outdoor yoga class in Times Square with several other teachers. As I took my seat on the stage and looked out at the sea of six thousand faces, it felt like an intimate gathering consisting of every age, race, and gender. I didn't expect such calm unity. At the end of the class, when everybody in the crowd had finished a beautiful collective *om*, I turned around and looked up the street. I could see the giant Marriott Marquis Hotel that now sits at the corner of Broadway and Forty-Fifth Street. It was the very corner where the Piccadilly Hotel had been—and where I'd spent those miserable yet life-changing days so long ago. Here I was, three blocks, thirty-five years, and a miraculous yogic mile from my former, confused, and desperate self.

Yoga Sequence:
Observing and Letting Go of Habits

One day, a twenty-six-year-old girl who I knew was in recovery came to class. I could see the tension in her jaw and the restlessness in her legs that indicate internal tension, struggle, and a yearning to run away. I've felt these symptoms in myself and recognize them in others who are dealing with addiction.

Yoga can be a powerful tool for addressing addiction. Habits or addictions often provide relief from feelings (physiological or emotional) that we're running from. In our yoga practice, we learn how to sit with sensations, emotions, stories, and learn that we don't have to react.

This balancing sequence is for everyone who is struggling with any habit, addiction, or just plain agitation or restlessness. It opens the hips and eases tension and restlessness in the jaw and legs, a few of the places we hold emotional obstructions, as well as our fight-or-flight impulses. We'll do the poses in vinyasa style in which each posture moves smoothly into the next, linked by breath.

Recovering addicts need to stand proudly and understand they may be the bravest people in the room. To be doing shavasana on a mat rather than lying in a ditch is to have the fortitude to climb a very steep mountain.

At the end of the class, I watched the woman in Final Relaxation. I saw that her eyes were still darting nervously, so I went over and gently but firmly held her feet. Quietly, she started to cry. A dam had broken, and the energy that had been blocked in her body was set free. I watched her jaw relax and her legs surrender. This was the release she needed.

Yoga teachers often think of hip-opening poses as merely external rotation and abduction, as in Full Lotus (padmasana) or Bound Angle Pose (baddha konasana). In this sequence, my goal is to find the expansive space in the entire circumference of the hip socket, which is relief.

Easy Pose (sukhasana). Sit with shins crossed, left in front of right (a). Exhale and fold your torso forward over your legs into **Easy Pose with Forward Bend** (b). Hold for 5 breaths. Inhale, lift up, and swing your left leg straight back behind your pelvis.

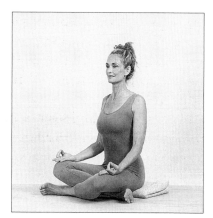

Easy Pose (a)

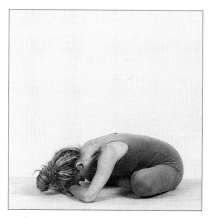

Easy Pose with Forward Bend (b)

Modified One-Legged King Pigeon (eka pada raja kapotasana). Position your right heel just in front of your left hip, with your right knee just a little outside the line of the right side of your hip. Align the front of your pelvis as parallel as possible to the front of your sticky mat. Support your raised torso by pressing your hands into the floor (a). Walk your hands forward, release your neck and head, and hold for 5 breaths (b). Then move your right leg back, tuck your back toes under, and move into **Downward-Facing Dog** (c). Pedal your legs one at a time for 30 seconds to a minute. Then set your knees on the floor, cross your shins, right in front of left, and repeat Easy Pose, Cross-Legged Forward Bend, and One-Legged King Pigeon on the opposite side, ending in Downward-Facing Dog.

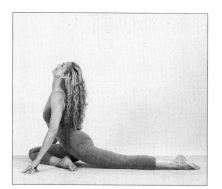

Modified One-Legged King Pigeon with Backbend (a)

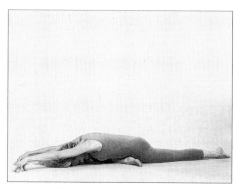

One-Legged King Pigeon with Forward Bend (b)

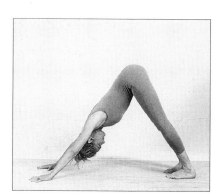

Downward-Facing Dog (c)

Seated Spinal Twist (ardha matsyendrasana). From Downward-Facing Dog, step your right foot forward into a lunge and slide your left knee to the floor outside of your right foot. Sit down between your heels (if your buttocks don't rest comfortably on the floor, use a block for support) with your right foot pressing firmly on the floor to the outside of the left thigh. Turn to the right and wrap your left arm around the right leg, hugging the thigh to your belly in **Seated Spinal Twist** (a). Hold for 5 breaths and then lower your right knee toward the floor, positioning your ankle just outside your left knee and come into **Ankle over Knee Pose (svastikasana)** (b). If this position is too difficult, sit in Easy Pose. Stay forward for 5 breaths. Then inhale, bring the torso up to sitting, slide your right foot off your left knee, and press the soles of your feet together, knees to the floor, in **Bound Angle Pose** (c). Hold for a few breaths, then lift your knees together, put your feet on the floor, and push up into **Wide-Knee Squat (malasana)** (d). Touch your inner feet together (or position them as closely together as you can manage), widen your knees, and drape your body forward between your legs for 5 breaths. Then lift your hips and slowly straighten your legs into **Standing Forward Bend** (e), knees straight, kneecaps actively pulled up toward the pelvis. If your hamstrings are tight or if there is strain in your lower back, bend your knees slightly. Hold for 5 breaths and walk back to **Downward-Facing Dog** (f). Repeat these six poses on the second side starting with Seated Spinal Twist. Come to stand in **Mountain Pose** (g).

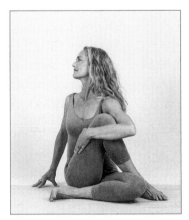
Seated Spinal Twist (a)

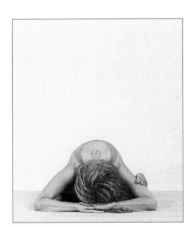
Ankle over Knee Pose
with a Forward Bend (b)

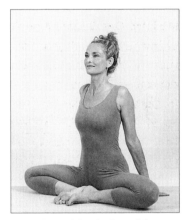
Bound Angle Pose (c)

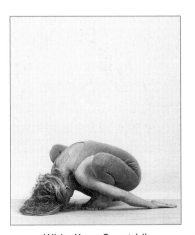
Wide-Knee Squat (d)

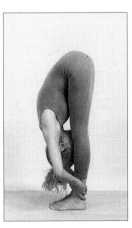
Standing Forward Bend (e)

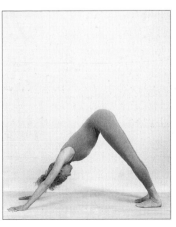
Downward-Facing Dog (f)

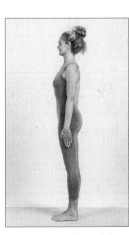
Mountain Pose (g)

Lord of the Dance Preparation (natarajasana). Bend your right knee, grip your right ankle with the right hand, and draw your heel as close to your buttock as possible, knee pointed to the floor. This will release your quadriceps and your psoas muscle. Stretch your left arm up. Open and close your jaw and move it side to side. Hold for 5 breaths. Switch sides. When both feet are back on the floor, take a wide step out to the right.

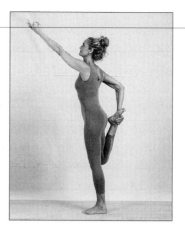

Lord of the Dance Preparation

Warrior II (virabhadrasana II). Turn your left toes in 15 degrees, your right toes out 90 degrees. Inhale with your arms parallel to the floor and bend your right knee to 90 degrees, making sure to position it over the ankle. Chant *om* 3 times to keep your mind focused and your jaw supple. Repeat on the opposite side, chant *om* again, then walk your feet together and step to the front of your mat. Warrior poses promote courage and strength.

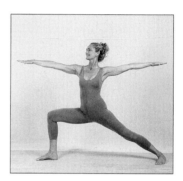

Warrior II

Mountain Pose with Lion Pose, face only (tadasana with simhasana). Stand in Mountain Pose, then bend your knees slightly and press your hands on your thighs. Open your mouth and roar like a lion, sticking out your tongue to release tension in your jaw and pent-up energy in your belly. Repeat 3 times. Lion Pose has a host of beneficial effects, such as stimulation of the thyroid and improved blood circulation. It has always helped me roar away shame and other emotional stagnation.

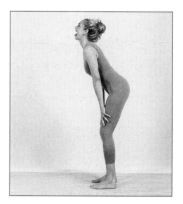

Mountain Pose with Lion

Sun Salutation A (surya namaskar A). Stand in **Mountain Pose** (a), then inhale and reach your arms overhead (b). Exhale into **Standing Forward Bend** (c). Inhale, bend your knees, and look forward; exhale, step or jump back to **Four-Limbed Staff Pose (chaturanga dandasana)** (d). If it isn't possible for you to support yourself resting only on your hands and balls of the feet, bend your knees to the floor, then flip to the tops of your feet, and on an inhale, move your chest through your arms into **Upward-Facing Dog** (e), then exhale to **Downward-Facing Dog** (f). Focus your mind on 5 cycles of breath. At the end of 5 breaths, bend your knees and walk or jump forward to **Standing Forward Bend** (g). Inhale, lift your arms up into a **Reverse Swan** (h), and come back to **Mountain Pose** (i). Repeat Sun Salutation A 3 to 5 times. The rhythm of this sequence is important and helps to calm the nervous system. After the final sequence, stay in Downward-Facing Dog, then lower your knees to the floor.

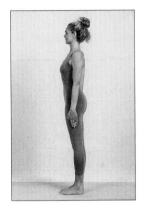

Sun Salutation A Mountain Pose (a)

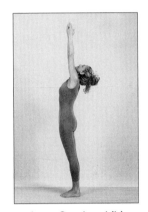

Arms Overhead (b)

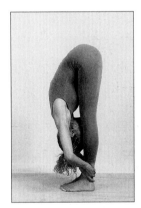

Standing Forward Bend (c)

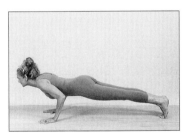

Four-Limbed Staff Pose (d)

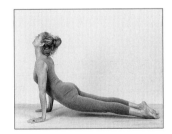

Upward-Facing Dog (e)

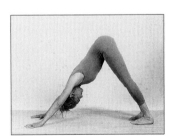

Downward-Facing Dog (f)

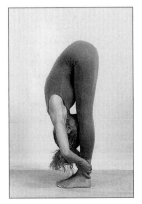

Standing Forward Bend (g)

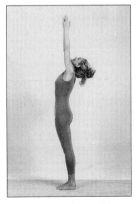

Reverse Swan (h)

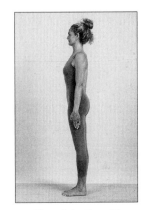

Mountain Pose (i)

Hero Pose (virasana). Bring your knees together and sit back between your feet (if your hips don't come to the floor, sit on a block). Stay for 5 breaths and make a buzzing sound like a bee on your exhale, creating a vibration in your jaw. Cross your shins and sit down behind your feet.

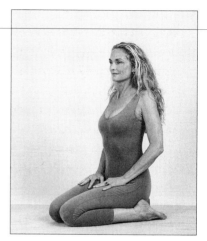

Hero Pose

Reverse Tabletop (purvottanasana). With your knees bent and your feet and buttocks on the floor, place your hands six inches behind you. Then inhale and lift your buttocks and torso as high as you can into Reverse Tabletop. Keep your head in a relatively neutral position. Lower down with an inhale, then lift up and lower down twice more. Sit back into . . .

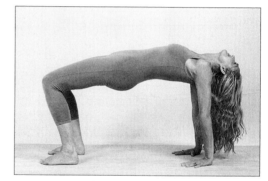

Reverse Tabletop

Easy Pose (sukhasana). Sit with your shins crossed, left in front of right, and perform **Shining Skull (kapalabhati),** a cleansing practice (*kriya*) that serves as a preparation for conscious breathing (*pranayama*). Breathe in only through your nose; each exhale will be a sharp burst, with the inhale a passive "rebound." Repeat rhythmically for 3 rounds, doing 9 cycles of Shining Skull. Take 3 natural breaths between rounds. Then lie down on your back.

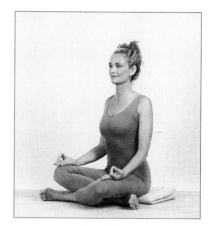

Easy Pose

Final Relaxation (shavasana). Strap your legs mid-thigh with a belt and place a weight on the top of your thighs. (If someone is antsy, sandbags or weights on the thighs can be calming.) Use an eye pillow to still darting eyes. Open and close your mouth and wiggle your jaw or massage it. Place your arms alongside your body, palms facing up. If your eyes continue to move restlessly under the closed lids, and/or if your breath becomes rapid, remove the weight and eye pillow. Stay in the pose for 7 minutes. If anxiousness persists, sit up in cross-legged meditation.

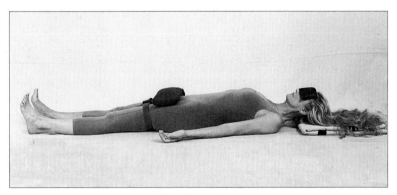

Final Relaxation

Yoga gives us a community, but it also gives us a link to our true selves (call it our soul, or our spirit). It is this connection that brings us to the innate beauty and love that our cravings obscure. In addition to working on our addictive habits one day at a time, we can work on them one pose at a time.

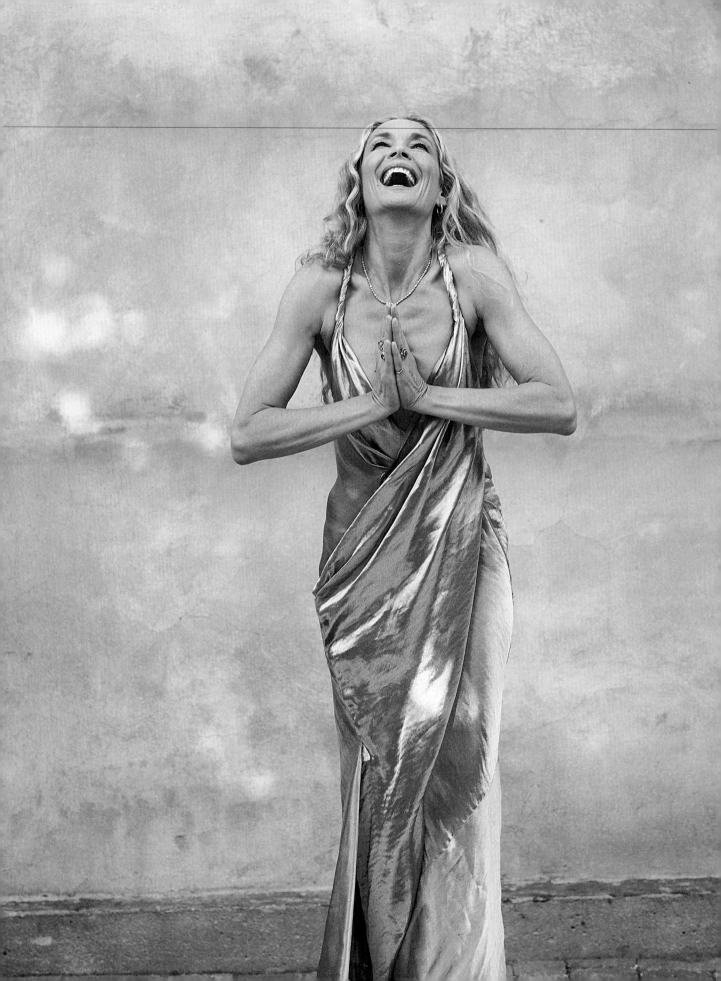

Chapter 4

FORGIVENESS

Forgiveness is part of the treasure you need
To craft your falcon wings
And return
To your true realm of
Divine freedom.
—"Forgiveness Is the Cash," Hafiz (tr. Ladinsky)

I'm not sure how I made it to this point in my life. Call it chance, fate, karma, or a guardian angel, but there seem to be too many instances of being in the right place at the right time for what happened to be just luck. We're all thrown different balls in life, and where we end up is a matter of which ones we pick up and run with.

After getting off heroin at the Piccadilly Hotel, my practical instincts kicked in. I needed a job.

I started searching the employment ads. One day, as I was walking up Madison Avenue, I passed a hotel called the Executive at Thirty-Eighth Street with a "Waitress Wanted" sign in the window. I went in but didn't see a restaurant. The man behind the desk told me to go outside and down the stairs to the left. You would have never known it was a restaurant if someone hadn't told you. When I entered, it was so dark I had to let my eyes adjust. Before I could make out any images, I heard a woman playing the piano and singing the blues. A couple of guys straight out of *The Godfather* were standing by the bar. The name of the restaurant was A Quiet Little Table in the Corner.

The manager hired me on the spot and handed me the uniform: a black leotard and fishnet stockings. It took him only a couple of days to see that I was a lousy waitress, so he made me the coat-check girl.

The restaurant attracted an eclectic crowd. Every booth had privacy curtains made of beads, as well as two light switches: the green light switch was for service, and the red one was to signal that the customers didn't want to be disturbed. Greta Garbo used to come in frequently for dinner. The man who brought her never sat down and always waited near the door. She was just like her character in *Grand Hotel*—"I want to be alone"—and nobody ever disturbed her. Garbo would order French onion soup and pay her bill with exact change, which she carefully counted out and left on the table.

Shortly after I started, a dark-haired man with a European accent walked in. He looked me up and down and, when I took his coat, he reached into his pocket and pulled out a business card. "My name is Zoli," he said. "You could be a model. Why don't you give me a call?"

I was suspicious, of course: some pretty bizarre things had already happened in the short time I'd been at the restaurant. One day, a man had offered me ten thousand dollars to let him watch me take a shower in nothing but high heels. The guy was a regular customer, but although I believed this would be a "hands-off" voyeuristic event and I needed money, I didn't go there.

Zoli's address was a brownstone on the Upper East Side. The office walls had pictures of real fashion models and a round table where professional bookers sat and worked with a giant Rolodex. Phones rang, the Rolodex spun, and deals were made. Mainly an agency for male models, it had a few women as well: Veruschka was on the Zoli roster at the time, as was Geena Davis, before she became an actress.

I felt like some Midwestern farm girl in Zoli's office, which, of course, I was, but where I came from didn't matter to them. The important thing was that I was 5 foot 9½ inches tall, 125 pounds, and had long legs. After talking to me for a few minutes, Zoli invited me to join the agency.

As I was leaving the office, one of his assistants walked me to the door. "How old are you?" he asked.

"Nineteen," I said.

"What year were you born?"

"1959."

"Let's make that 1962," he suggested. "You're sixteen now." He winked, I smiled, and that was that. The message was clear: at nineteen, I was already too old.

For the next twenty-one years, I lied about my age, even to my best model friends. Whenever I was booked for a job abroad, I was always terrified that someone—the photographer, the other models, the client—would see my passport, and I'd be caught, fired from the booking, and mortified.

The bookers started sending me out on "go-see's" to photographers in order to pose for "test shots" to build my portfolio. This was the first step. Though these weren't paying gigs, they were still exciting—and scary.

Jeff and I had moved into the basement of my uncle's house in Danbury, Connecticut, since we couldn't afford an apartment in New York City. I took the train into the city every day and pounded the pavement. I never missed a go-see. I didn't feel like model material, but I kept showing up. A model eventually wants a book full of editorial tear sheets—photographs that appear in magazines—rather than test shots or catalogue shots. It was going to take me a while: for every thirty to fifty castings I went on, I probably got one callback.

Gradually, though, the go-sees led to bookings. One of my first jobs was posing for romance-novel covers. The client paid $75 an hour, half the going rate. The studio where we did the shoot was a tiny fourth-floor walkup that resembled the greenroom of a strip club. The photographer was at least eighty years old—a real character and passionate about her work. The clothes she gave me to wear were dirty and looked as if they might have come from a high school drama wardrobe. Fortunately, we were selling sexy books, not clothes, and I was usually posing in the arms of big, muscle-bound male models like Fabio. My job was to muster some semblance of cleavage in a white, ruffled, off-the-shoulder blouse while affecting a look of raw desire. We could usually shoot three covers in an hour.

One day the agency called with big news: the J. C. Penney catalogue had booked me for a cover try. I was more excited about this booking than any in my career—which would include shoots for *Cosmopolitan*, *Harper's Bazaar*, *Glamour*, and *Vogue*. Where I grew up, the Penney's catalogue *was* fashion, and J. C. Penney the fanciest store in Bluffton. None of my New York friends could have understood J. C. Penney's significance to a girl from Bluffton, Indiana. To say we were a little behind in the fashion arena was an understatement. I kept my excitement to myself so as not to appear uncool.

When you're booked for a cover try, it's exactly that—a try. There are no guarantees. Penney's did end up using me on the cover of its catalogue, wearing a red blazer, a white shirt, and a loose black tie with jeans—a hip, boyfriend kind of look. When the catalogue came out, it was proudly displayed in the J. C. Penney store on Market Street in Bluffton. Mom and Dad were relieved I was working and bursting with pride. I was making $150 an hour.

In high school, I had come across a want ad in the Fort Wayne newspaper for a modeling agency that I cut out and read over and over. It said that if a girl was 5 foot 9 inches or taller, weighed 120 pounds, and had wide-set eyes, she could be a model. That was me! I'd never thought of myself as pretty. Growing up, I was always the flat-chested girl my brothers teased. They'd taunt me, "Colleen, stand sideways and stick out your tongue. You'll look like a zipper!"

When I was sixteen years old, I met a photographer who lived in Decatur, a town near Bluffton, who wanted to take some photographs of me. Even though I was clumsy and shy, I felt comfortable in front of the camera. I could move and strike poses that looked good on film. It was almost as if I'd done it in a past life.

Something in me from an early age loved to find expression through my body. I wonder if that in itself would have pointed me to a modeling career. Would I have become a model if Zoli hadn't stopped by the restaurant? Even getting the break I did, what were the odds that I would succeed?

Some people believe we make our own luck. I prefer the yoga and Buddhist perspective: What seems like good luck, or good karma, in one moment, can easily turn into bad luck, or bad karma, the next moment. Conversely, bad luck can result in something good. In yoga, we learn that there's no such thing as "good" or "bad," because everything is always in flux and rarely what it seems. The key is not to get attached to any one scenario or outcome. One of my favorite Zen stories captures this perfectly.

For many years, an old farmer had worked his fields with a loyal horse. One day, the horse ran away. Upon hearing the news, the farmer's neighbors stopped by to commiserate: "Such bad luck!" they said to the farmer.

"Maybe," he replied.

The next morning the horse showed up, bringing with it three wild horses.

"How wonderful!" the neighbors exclaimed. "You have three new horses!"

"Maybe," replied the farmer.

The following day, the farmer's son tried to ride one of the untamed horses. He was thrown and broke his leg. The neighbors came to offer their condolences.

"Such terrible news!" they said.

"Maybe," answered the farmer.

The next day, military officers showed up at the village to draft all the young men into the army. Since the farmer's son's leg was broken, they rejected him. The neighbors congratulated the farmer on how the accident had benefited his family.

"Maybe," he said.

And so it goes. Life is sometimes beautiful, sometimes ugly, sometimes sad, sometimes joyful. It's a wild, unpredictable ride. The best we can do is to take the ride with love and a sense of humor. Notice your breath in the present moment, whether you consider it to be a "good" moment or "bad" moment. Because that moment is all we have, and as my dad always says, "This too shall pass."

In the early days of my modeling career—before cell phones became the norm—I kept my telephone numbers and appointments in a Filofax. By then, Jeff and I had rented a small apartment in White Plains, still north of the city but closer than Danbury, from where I commuted every day. Because we were supposed to stay in contact with the agency, my "office" was a phone booth at Grand Central Station, and I'd call in from there for my next day's go-sees. Jeff and I had so little money that I walked everywhere; taking the subway was a luxury. I planned my routes carefully so I could pass the vendors of my favorite cheap food: pizza, pretzels, and black-and-white cookies.

One day, my agent, Liza, told me that I had been booked for a go-see with a photographer named Robin Saidman who wanted to do some test shots. I had seen one of Robin Saidman's spreads in *Glamour*. The pictures were stunning. I was excited to meet this Robin, whom I assumed was a woman. When I arrived at the studio, though, a rock-star-handsome man opened the door.

"I'm here to see Robin," I said.

"Ah," he replied in a gorgeous British accent. "That would be me."

I had never met a man named Robin, and we laughed about my confusion. He was from a small town south of London, had puppy-dog eyes, and was wickedly funny and charming. He was also incredibly smart, with two degrees from the University of Edinburgh in Scotland and one from the Royal College of Art in London.

Robin put me on hold for a shoot with *Company* magazine, England's version of *Glamour*. If I got it, the assignment would move me to the next level of models. I called in every day to check with Liza, my booker. "Nope," she'd answer. "It's still tentative." But one day I called in and she said: "They've confirmed. You'll be going to a village off the coast of Crete to shoot a ten-page spread, plus the cover."

I had no idea where Crete was, but I was delirious with excitement. I'd never been on an airplane before. Frantically, I made arrangements to get a passport, and two weeks later I was on a flight to the Aegean. Lefkara was the name of the village where we did the shoot, and to this day I've never seen a more exquisite place. We were there for a week, and it felt as if we'd been transported back in time. The streets were cobblestone, and beautiful girls and women sat on benches in the town square, making the lace the village is famous for. Joy seemed imprinted on the faces of everyone in Lefkara, from the children to the elderly women carrying their bread and vegetables home from the market. The open-air market held rows of glistening fish caught just hours before. Growing up in Indiana, the only seafood I'd ever eaten was Mrs. Paul's frozen fish sticks, which my mom served every Friday.

The shoot went well, although I felt a lot of insecurity. My "look" was very natural—casual clothes, very little makeup, lace woven into my wavy hair. Robin wanted me to just *be* in the situation—to act as naturally as possible. I tried to pose. Suddenly I had to learn a new way to relate to the camera. Over the next twenty years, I would spend hundreds of hours in front of Robin's lens, and it was never easy. He demanded that I be real, which felt very uncomfortable. And yet it stretched me.

This was one of my first lessons in human *being* rather than human *doing*. I had to be in the moment rather than hiding behind an artificial identity. Robin wanted to photograph *me*, not some model I was pretending to be. The problem was I didn't know who "me" was. Nisargadatta dedicated a whole book to this topic: *I Am That*. He writes, "Give up all questions except one, 'Who am I?' After all, the only fact you are sure of is that you 'are.' The 'I am' is certain, the 'I am this' is not. Struggle to find out what you are in reality."

The practice of yoga helps us get to the heart of the question *Who am I?* Am I my personality? Am I my career? Am I my body? Am I my emotions? Nisargadatta says that identifying so strongly with self-created labels such as personality, career, body, and emotions keeps us separated from who we really are. When we pare away all that we are not, what are we left with . . . our true essence? Discovering our essence is liberating because we experience the self as whole, not separate. In that state, there is absolute love without fear.

Serious stuff, and I'm still digging into the questions: *Who am I? Who am I not?* I've gotten glimpses of "no separation" in *shavasana*, meditation, and *pranayama*—even while folding laundry or listening to music. I've experienced moments of expanse, of no desperation or alienation, of stepping back and watching my thoughts and breath. Robin was asking me to shed a layer of pretense. Ultimately, this brings about a state of relaxation in the present moment. Propping up an identity, it turns out, takes a lot of effort.

After the *Company* shoot, Zoli advised me to relocate to Paris for a few months to build up my tear sheets, which are the editorial and advertising jobs that appear in print. At the time, there was a lot of editorial work in Paris, and the photographers loved American girls. I felt bad about being away from Jeff, but the truth was we were already living very different lives.

I moved into a flat that was the servants' quarters of a fancy Parisian apartment off the Champs Élysées with five other girls, including my roommate, Julie Hannahan, who became my best friend. The other four girls didn't seem to be doing much modeling; on weekends they would go out on a fancy yacht that was owned by a wealthy Middle Easterner and come back with fistfuls of cash. Julie and I never accepted the "weekend yacht" invitation.

In Paris, I didn't experience the glamorous clichés of the "model's life"—making tons of money, dressing in designer clothes, going to fancy restaurants and clubs, and having a chauffeur. In reality, the American models in Paris worked their butts off for very little money and hung out at the McDonald's on the Champs Élysées every evening after work. Most of my meals were a large order of fries and a chocolate milk shake. The daily grind meant getting up and going on castings or bookings, meeting at McDonald's, hanging out with Julie, and being homesick. Mostly, I was feeling distant and estranged from Jeff and not sure where I belonged. Still, it was worth it, because when I returned to New York midway through 1981, I had a decent portfolio of editorial tear sheets from magazines including *Elle* and *Madame Figaro*. I began to get regular work.

As the Zen story goes, opportunities can come along that at first appear auspicious, then turn into something very different. I was booked for what seemed like a great assignment: a three-day shoot in the tropics at $1,200 a day. The job was for a reputable catalogue; I knew both the photographer and the art director, with whom I'd worked before.

I flew down, and the photographer picked me up at the airport. He greeted me warmly and said he'd take me to the hotel so that I could rest before the shoot. Instead, he drove me to a nondescript building. We climbed the stairs to a cinder-block room with yellow walls and two twin beds. The art director was standing there with a strange look on his face. Something was seriously wrong.

Inside, I felt panic, but on the outside, I managed to stay cool. I thanked the photographer for meeting me at the airport and said I would take a nap. I suggested the two men go back to their hotel and we would meet later. I sat down on the bed, at which point the photographer climbed on top of me and started kissing me, while the art director leered, looking eager to get in on the action.

I managed to get the photographer to stop and then turned to the art director.

"Look, I know you're married," I said. "I know you have children. How would your wife feel if she knew what you're doing? And how would you feel if this were happening to your daughter? Take me back to the airport, and I'll forget this ever happened. I won't tell anyone." It must have struck a chord, because they muttered to each other, and the art director drove me to the airport, where I slept on the floor of the terminal until I could get a flight home.

When my plane landed in New York, I called Jeff and asked him to come get me. I was numb. I couldn't talk, except to say that I needed to go home to my family. He drove me home. Jeff was confused and angry. I was sad and lonely and knew our marriage wasn't going to last.

My stay was the respite I needed. The house was bright and cheerful. Dad was working days; Ed and John were the only kids left at home, and since both were musicians, music was always playing. I slept a lot and tried to make sense of what had happened. Had I done something to elicit it? Had I been flirtatious on the casting call? Had I dressed too suggestively?

At the time, I blamed myself for the photo-shoot situation and didn't want to confront or relive what had happened. The right thing would have been for me to tell the agency what had gone down and let the art director and photographer deal with the consequences. But "right" action isn't always the easiest course. I felt similarly about my marriage. I wanted out but felt guilty about breaking a commitment and letting Jeff and his family down.

The roller coaster of my life was making me motion sick: the pain that I'd caused my family, the scare at the photo shoot, and the dissolution of my marriage. I didn't know then that in each instance I'd done the best I could at the time. Sometimes it's much easier to forgive another person than to forgive yourself.

Nisargadatta writes that loving oneself is the first step to being able to love another. But we have to know ourselves before we can love ourselves. With love comes self-respect and gratitude. With self-respect and gratitude come clarity and "right action." To develop this love takes practice. Yoga, breath work, meditation, and study of yoga scriptures are practices that can open the door to knowledge and love—of ourselves and others.

The ending of Jeff's and my marriage was painful and ugly. I returned to New York and moved in with a model named Jacky Fuller. Jeff closed up our apartment in White Plains and moved back to the Midwest. I got paid for the bogus catalogue job and didn't say a word about it until many years later.

My parents had always been supportive of me. Now I was in a position to do something for them. My dad loved antique cars, and his dream car was a white 1952 MG with red leather interiors. My brother Mark found the car, I bought it, and my sister Peggy hid it in her garage. In December, I flew home for the holidays and we all gathered at Peggy's on Christmas morning for her traditional egg casserole. Mark pulled out an encyclopedia of cars and casually asked Dad to pick out the one he liked best. He pointed to the MG.

We were all trying to act nonchalant. "Hey, Dad," Mark said, "why don't we go out to the garage for a minute?" When they got there, we were all standing around the car, grinning.

"Merry Christmas, Dad," I said.

At first, he didn't say a word. "What is this?" he asked.

"Your Christmas present," I answered.

Mark opened the driver's door so Dad could get in, but he was still stunned. He turned to me.

"Honey, you can't do this."

"Yes, I can, Dad."

The tears we all shed that morning felt like a rain shower clearing away emotional dirt and debris. I could feel the tension and guilt I'd been carrying for so long start to dissolve. The sky was clearing. I was back in the family, and forgiven. And I forgave myself.

Dad took impeccable care of the MG and drove it around Bluffton for years. I like to imagine that every time he put on his Italian cap and sat down in the red leather seats with Mom at his side, he smiled and thought about his prodigal daughter who returned home bearing gifts for her beloved parents.

Yoga Sequence: Loving-Kindness Toward Ourselves

Yoga teachers see it all. We recognize ourselves in our students, which is why we say that our students are our teachers. There's the student who comes up after every class with a new "woe is me" story. There's the student who seems so uninterested you're not sure why he comes at all. Then there's the bald student who's finishing chemotherapy, her body still emanating the metallic smell of chemo. She has the brightest smile and says, "I'm so grateful for this practice."

Some of our problems are self-inflicted, some aren't. Either way, we don't want pain, guilt, and anger to shut us down. This sequence wrings out the emotions that create obstacles and lack of internal space in our bodies. Yoga increases flexibility and range of motion, but its real work is to create a deeper sense of centeredness and ease within. Someone can have tight muscles and a spacious inner world; another can be flexible yet bound up internally. Yoga clears the body, so we have enough space to bear all our experiences.

Dishonesty and blame will keep the body locked up. Honesty and forgiveness allow you to live fully in the present moment.

Not forgiving someone is like eating rat poison and wishing the other person would die. You may be able to pinpoint where you hold lack of forgiveness in your body. For me, it's my throat. You can address areas with yoga and gain temporary relief, but if you don't forgive, the opening will be superficial.

This sequence is about letting go and learning to ride the waves. We are coaxing the body to open, but we are not insisting. Use the twists to open places that may be harboring "stuck" feelings, such as the pelvis, belly, diaphragm, or throat. Use the backbends to open your heart to compassion toward yourself and others.

The first time you do this practice, take your hands to prayer position and dedicate your practice to someone you love dearly who makes your insides light up with love. The second time, dedicate it to someone toward whom you are fairly neutral. The third time, dedicate it to someone from whom you want to ask forgiveness or whom you need to forgive. Notice where your body clenches. If it is too difficult to dedicate your practice to that person, let it go and come back to it on another day. Once you have made your dedication, chant *om* three times, creating a space that's safe, sacred, and free of judgment.

Start in **Bound Angle (baddha konasana)** with the soles of your feet together, knees wide (a). Then move into **Prone Restorative Twist (modified bharadvajasana)** by dropping your left knee over to the right side and placing the top of your left foot in the arch of your right. Pull one end of the bolster against your outer right hip, lay your torso over it, and turn your head to the left (b). Stay for 8 breaths, then turn your head to the right for 8 breaths (c). This should intensify the twist (if it's too intense, turn your head back to the first position). Change sides and repeat.

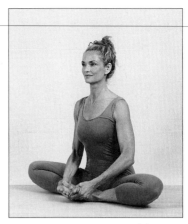

Bound Angle Pose (a)

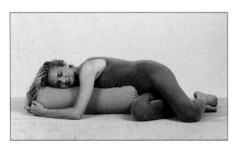

Prone Restorative Twist (b)

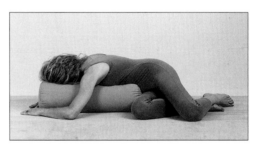

Prone Restorative Twist (c)

Seated Simple Twist (bharadvajasana). Come back to Bound Angle Pose. Drop your left knee over to the right side and place the top of your left foot in the arch of your right. Twist to the right, with your hands on the floor outside the right thigh, and then repeat on the left side. Stay in the pose for 5 breaths on each side. In each twist, focus on the feeling of "wringing out" all the way from your feet, up your legs, into your pelvis, then through the lower, middle, and upper back into your neck and head. Feel the twist as a pump that squeezes and releases. Make small movements in and out of the twist several times.

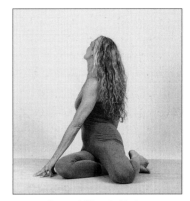

Seated Simple Twist

Bent-Knee Seated Twist C (marichyasana C). Start in Staff Pose (dandasana), legs extended forward, torso held upright. Then fold your left knee deeply and set your foot in front of your left sit bone. Twist to the left and hug your left knee with your right arm, turning your head to the left. Gently rock in and out of the pose for 5 breaths on each side. Repeat on the other side.

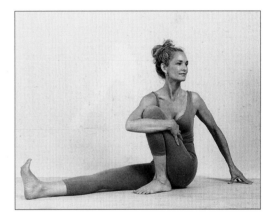

Bent-Knee Seated Twist C

Bent-Knee Seated Twist A (marichyasana A). Return to Staff Pose, bend your right knee deeply, and set your foot in front of your right sit bone. Take your right elbow to the inside of your right knee and twist to the left. Root your legs into the floor and float your chest like a helium balloon. Hold for 5 easy breaths and repeat on the other side.

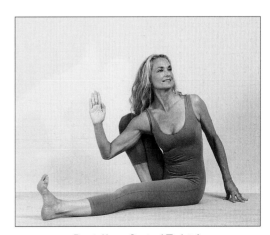

Bent-Knee Seated Twist A

Shift onto your hands and knees, tuck your toes under, and lift your hips into **Downward-Facing Dog (adho mukha shvanasana)** (a), keeping your knees bent, for 5 breaths. Focus on straightening your arms and moving your hips back. Then straighten your legs for 5 more breaths. Come down to your hands and knees, and while resting there, slide your right arm underneath your left arm and drop your right shoulder and right side of your face to the floor into **Thread the Needle Pose** (b). Use the press of your left fingertips to control how deeply you twist. Hold the pose for 5 breaths and change sides. Lift into **Downward-Facing Dog** (c), then drop your right knee to the floor and roll to the inside of the left foot, keeping the left leg straight. Lift your left arm toward the ceiling in **Modified Side Plank (modified vasishthasana)** (d). Hold for 5 breaths, repeat on the opposite side, and return to **Downward-Facing Dog** (e).

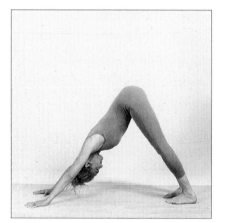
Downward-Facing Dog (a)

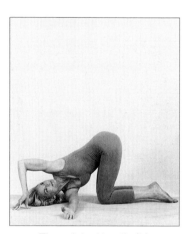
Thread the Needle (b)

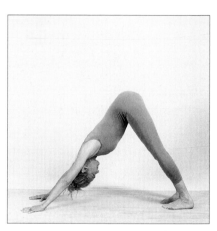
Downward-Facing Dog (c)

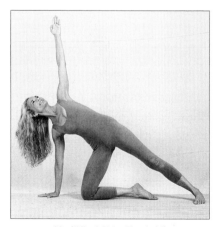
Modified Side Plank (d)

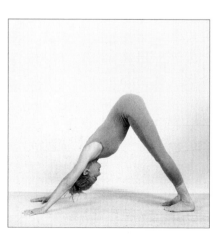
Downward-Facing Dog (e)

Modified Revolved Side Angle (modified parivritta parshvakonasana). From Downward-Facing Dog, step your left foot forward and, keeping your right hand on the floor, press your left thumb into your outer left hip crease, pulling the hip back and down. Reach strongly through the back leg and twist your upper body to the left (a). Return to **Downward-Facing Dog** (b). Repeat on the other side, holding the pose for 5 breaths.

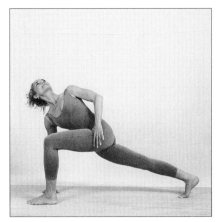

Modified Revolved Side Angle Pose (a)

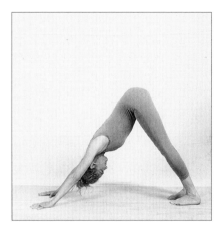

Downward-Facing Dog (b)

Sit down with your legs forward in **Staff Pose** (a). Then bend your left knee and open it out to the side into **Revolved Bent-Knee Seated Forward Bend (parivritta janu shirshasana),** your shin angled to slightly more than 90 degrees (b). Lower your right elbow and forearm, palm facing up, to the inside of your right leg and stretch your left arm over your left ear. Lean back and twist to the left. Hold for 5 breaths and repeat on the other side.

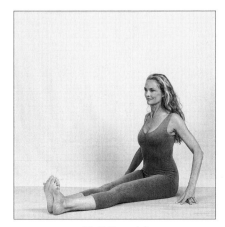

Staff Pose (a)

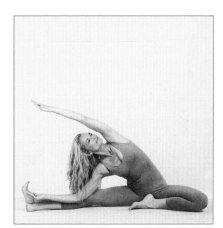

Revolved Bent-Knee Seated
Forward Bend (b)

Supported Fish Pose (matsyasana). Lie faceup on your bolster (or rolled-up blankets), its long axis perpendicular to your spine. The shoulder blades should be firmly supported and the head resting comfortably either on the floor or a thickly folded blanket. Stretch your arms out to the side, elbows bent like a cactus. Stay for 15 breaths.

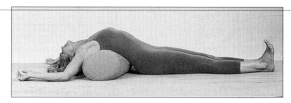

Supported Fish Pose

Cobra Pose (bhujangasana). Lie on your mat facedown. Press your hands to the floor on either side of your chest. Then pull your waist long and lift your upper chest with an inhale into Cobra. Hold for a few breaths, then lower back down on an exhale. Repeat 3 times.

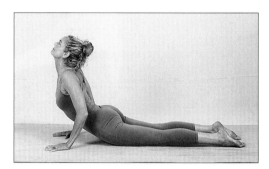

Cobra Pose

Bridge Pose (setu bandhasana). Lie on your back, with your knees bent and your feet on the floor, heels just in front of your sit bones. Lift your hips on an inhale, interlace your fingers underneath your pelvis, and press your arms into the floor. Hold for 5 breaths. Lower down, change the interlace of your fingers, and lift up again on the inhale. Stay for 5 breaths.

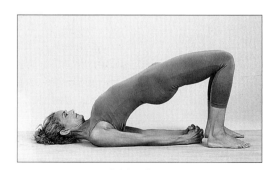

Bridge Pose

Legs Up the Wall (viparita karani mudra). Place your bolster parallel to and about 4 to 6 inches from a wall (closer if you are short, farther if you are tall). Sit on the bolster with one hip against the wall. Exhale and swing around, shoulders on the floor, legs up the wall (a). You may slide off the bolster, so try to keep your buttocks as close to the wall as possible. Ideally, your sit bones will drop down into the space between the bolster and the wall, giving your front torso a smooth, rounded shape. If the shape seems flat or hollow, bend your knees, press your feet to the wall, lift your hips, and slide the bolster an inch or two farther away from the wall. Then settle back down and check the shape of your torso again. If your hamstrings are tight, bend your knees slightly (b). Stay in the pose for 3 to 5 minutes, keeping your legs moderately active.

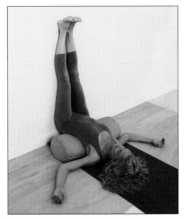

Legs Up the Wall (a)

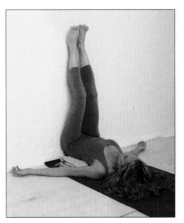

Legs Up the Wall Variation (b)

Final Relaxation (shavasana). Lie down on your back with legs straight and arms alongside the body in Final Relaxation for 3 to 5 minutes. Release all muscular effort and bathe in the beauty and love of the present moment.

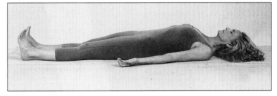

Final Relaxation

The Sufi poet Rumi wrote, "This being human is a guesthouse." We don't pick and choose who will show up, but we invite all to come inside as honorable guests— even anger and shame. He says we should meet them at the door, laughing like a perfect host. He advises us to be grateful for each guest; they have been sent as guides from beyond.

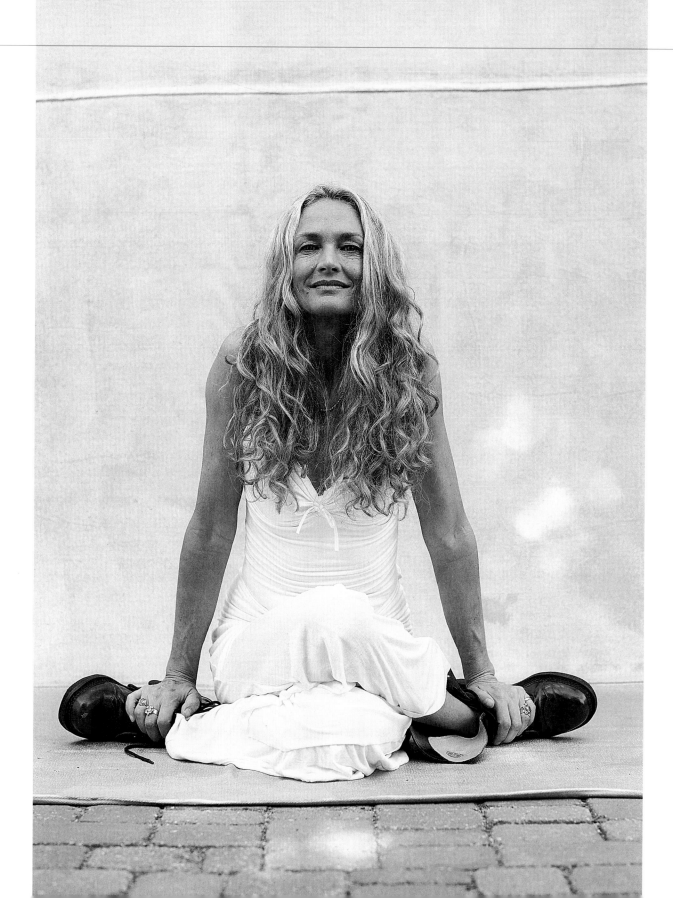

Chapter 5

CONFIDENCE

M[aharaj]: *"I am" is the ultimate fact. "Who am I?"*
is the ultimate question to which everybody must find an answer.
Q[uestioner]: *"The same answer?"*
M: *The same in essence, varied in expression.*

—*I Am That*, Nisargadatta Maharaj

After the *Company* shoot in Crete, I got a message from Zoli that the designer Valentino wanted to use me in an advertising campaign and I was to go to Milan on my way to Paris. The photographer would be Marco Glaviano, a famous name in the fashion world. I was excited and nervous. This would be my first big advertising job, a whole different ball game from the editorial booking for *Company*, which was great for my portfolio but didn't pay much. Advertising was far more lucrative and gave models greater exposure because the ads could appear on bus stops and billboards and in magazines.

When I got to the studio in Milan, one of the crew motioned for me to sit in a chair. Several stylists began circling me, looking at my long, curly, dirty blond hair and speaking in rapid-fire Italian. All of a sudden, one of them grabbed some scissors and began chopping. He cut my hair to chin length and dried it so that it was straight as a board. I was in shock. I loved my hair. Tears were streaming down my face, though no one seemed to notice or care. I looked in the mirror and didn't recognize the woman looking back at me. *Who was she?* She was sophisticated and classy, perfectly crafted for the elegant Valentino brand. Here I was in Milan, a model working for a fancy Italian designer, being shot by a top photographer. Isn't this what every model aspired to? We worked late into the night, and I began to embrace my short hair—and the new, dignified side of myself that I never even knew existed.

I had been in Paris a few months when the issue of *Company* magazine came out. There was my face, staring out from every newsstand in the city. It felt crazy, and even though I was proud, I also wanted to run and hide. One part of me wanted to tell everyone who walked by, "Hey! That's me on that magazine!" Another part wanted to buy up all the issues and throw them onto a bonfire. I was relieved that many of the other models felt the same way and had conflicted feelings of accomplishment and vulnerability. Throughout my career, no matter how beautiful the makeup, how elegant the clothes, how subtle and artistic the lighting was in my pictures, I would always see the awkward girl from Indiana.

My first six months in Paris in 1981 gave me a wider view of the modeling world. The week I arrived, designers were planning their upcoming couture shows and selecting models to walk the runway. I had no idea how to "walk," and every designer seemed to want something different. I watched other girls and tried to emulate their struts, but I wasn't very good at it. I walked on my toes. I was self-conscious. Basically, I walked like a tomboy straight out of the cornfields.

Two designers, Azzedine Alaïa and Kenzo, took a chance on me. They were the sweetest men in the world, and I loved their clothes. Kenzo's collection was fun and casual and he wanted his models to walk nonchalantly; Alaia's collection was as sexy and sophisticated as you can get, and he wanted us to swagger seductively. I had no feel for the runway and I couldn't do either walk, so those shows were the beginning and end of my catwalk career.

When I got back to New York, I had a decent portfolio. Anna Wintour, the future *Vogue* editor, was at the helm of *New York* magazine at the time and took a liking to me. She used me on several covers and in editorial spreads. I attribute much of my success to her belief in me. *Cosmopolitan* started to book me. My career was picking up steam, and I was making money.

With that momentum, I switched to Elite Model Management, a hipper, trendier agency known for getting its girls the best editorial jobs. I was assigned to a booker named Caroline Kramer, who took me under her wing and pushed me hard, treating every job I got as her own personal victory.

In 1983, I got a booking in Paris, and once again, my agent suggested I stay and take jobs that would update and strengthen my portfolio. I moved into a models' apartment right around the corner from our favorite McDonald's. I was much busier this time and started getting more prestigious jobs. Two top photographers, Claus Wickrath and Gilles Bensimon, started using me on a regular basis. Times were good. I worked like a dog.

Unlike at home, in Paris the agency weighed us regularly. They wanted me at 55 kilos—121.25 pounds—but with all the buttery croissants and McDonald's French fries, my weight shot up to 61 kilos, or 134.48 pounds. I started obsessing. Like all the girls, I would only get on the scale first thing in the morning after emptying my bladder and bowels. I'd remove my jewelry and stand there stark naked. Most of the seven other models in our apartment purged to control their weight. I probably would have done the same except I couldn't get my gag reflex to work. As a result, I had to be unbelievably disciplined about what I ate. One day, I even calculated the calories in a Tic Tac before popping it into my mouth.

Weight wasn't the only challenge. My eyes were usually puffy when I woke up and would stay that way for several hours. This would provoke mini-crises on my morning shoots. I never learned to speak French or Italian, but I became very familiar with the phrases for "bags under the eyes" in both languages. My stomach would sink when I heard photographers and stylists whispering the words *poches* and *borse*.

I tried to do everything to get rid of those bags. I put tea compresses and ice and cucumbers on my eyes. I spent hundreds of dollars on creams that didn't work. I avoided salt. I even tried to sleep sitting up so fluid wouldn't collect under the skin. Finally, I realized that the only way that I could look rested (i.e., no bags) was by *not* sleeping. Of course, this was ridiculous, unsustainable, and wreaked havoc on my mood and my health. But, if sleeping sitting up—or not sleeping at all—was what it took, I was going to do it.

I headed back to New York at the end of the year with a killer portfolio of European tear sheets and started to shoot for magazines such as *Harper's Bazaar* and *Glamour* with brilliant photographers including James Moore and Albert Watson. I bought an apartment on West Broadway. It was a wild, fast time in New York. Models were always on the invitation lists to the coolest nightclubs: Studio 54, Area, Limelight, and the Mudd Club. Drugs were everywhere—particularly cocaine. I had sworn off heroin, but I did occasionally smoke pot or do a line of cocaine when I went out.

One day, I was sent on a go-see with the legendary photographer Richard Avedon, who had photographed everyone—including the Beatles, Bob Dylan, Jackie Onassis, Marilyn Monroe, Andy Warhol, and Audrey Hepburn.

When I walked into his studio, Avedon was in the middle of a shoot for *Vogue* with a model named Gia Carangi, whose beauty literally took my breath away. She was raw and outrageous, but also shy and vulnerable. Everyone in the studio loved her. Gia was openly bisexual and flirted with me. I was flustered and flattered, and I could also see in her eyes and body language that she was high. One part of me wanted to do heroin with her—to curl up in her arms and let her know that I understood—but I didn't.

Sadly, Gia died of AIDS in 1986 when she was only twenty-six. She was one of the most beautiful women in the world and in a different league from me as a model. I always wished I'd known her better. As Maya Angelou said: "You remember people not by what they do, but by how they make you feel." Gia made me feel special.

◆　　◆　　◆

Over the years, yoga has helped me find perspective on many of the things I went through in the modeling world. Occasionally, I'm asked to speak to groups of young models. I tell them that if they want peace of mind, they need to develop what I would now call a yogic mind-set so that when things happen they'll be able to take them less personally. Of course, it's pretty challenging when a person's professional value is based entirely on her physical body; eventually, models start to believe that we are these "shells"—the specifications on our model cards. Along with the photo, mine was printed with these words: Height 5' 9½"; Bust 34, Waist 24, Hips 34; Shoes 9; Dress Size 4; Hair, honey-blond; Eyes, blue-green. One card added, "Excellent legs."

For a long time, I lived on an emotional seesaw, exhilarated if I got a booking and despondent if I didn't. I was obsessed with getting a Guess! jeans campaign—I don't know why I wanted it so badly, but I'd go to the annual casting and come home and recite Hail Marys as I listened to the messages on my answering machine. I never did get a Guess! campaign.

Another time I was on a modeling job in New Orleans and was angry that I was getting the shitty light and the shitty clothes compared to the other models on the shoot. I was sitting in the trailer eating peanut M&Ms and feeling sorry for myself. At one point I went into a bathroom in a nearby bar (I hated the tiny bathrooms in the motor home) and noticed a bumper sticker on the wall that said, "Life is 10 percent what happens to you and 90 percent how you respond to it." It was like getting hit with the stick by the Zen master: If I was wallowing in self-pity, then that was my choice.

Life is full of acceptance and rejection. Unfortunately, many of us focus on the rejection. Yoga tells us it's more useful to practice *swaha*, the idea of which is *do the best you can, and let go of the rest.* Tibetan Buddhists often translate *swaha* as "so be it." *Swaha* is the rudder that can help us maintain equilibrium.

◆ ◆ ◆

By 1987, I had reached the advanced age of twenty-eight. I was aging out of the "middle" level at my agency, but I wasn't quite ready for the "elite" division. One day, the agency asked me to come into the office for a meeting. After I sat down, I was very matter-of-factly told that it would be a good idea for me to get breast implants and to get my teeth capped so they would be whiter and bigger.

Models almost always do what we're told. The agency made an appointment for me with a dentist. As he explained the teeth-capping procedure—he was going to file my teeth down to small stubs and place permanent caps over them—I flashed back to Mom and Dad sitting at the dining-room table figuring out which bills to pay. My braces had been one of the expenses that took priority, and my mom had been incredibly proud of my teeth.

That was it. I didn't get my teeth or my tits done. Instead, I switched agencies and eventually found my way to the Ford Modeling Agency, which wasn't as sexy or trendy and didn't focus as much on the hip editorial jobs. At Ford, with my new bookers Jill Perlman and Patty Sinclair, I was proud to be reborn as a "catalogue queen."

And that's what I became best known for. Over the past thirty years I've worked for Chadwicks of Boston, Talbots, Sundance, Avon Fashion, Brownstone Studio, Spiegel, Saks Fifth Avenue, Macy's, Bloomingdale's, J. Jill, Roaman's, and Lane Bryant, among others. I always approached the jobs with the same respect and professionalism as I had for the top fashion magazines. Truthfully, I'm most proud of the work I did between the ages of forty-eight and fifty-two, which included nearly every Eileen Fisher campaign. In a culture that worships youth, I admire Eileen for embracing beauty in women my age. It sends a powerful message to the world. Eileen is a yogi herself. She told me she booked me because I was "in my body" and I "knew who I was."

Yoga Sequence: Strength and Courage
to Stand on Your Own Two Feet

All women, including models, yearn to discover their immense inner beauty and to find inspiration, as well as refuge, as gravity and time alter their outer bodies. Coming to a love of one's self takes discipline, diligence, and dedication—all keys to being a well-adjusted woman in this crazy world. I aspire for every one of us to be real, to look in the mirror and say, "*You are the bomb.*"

Models seem drawn to yoga in unusually high numbers. My guess is they come because yoga helps them find balance and a sense of self in a profession where outward appearances matter most. Most models have been on the roller coaster of acceptance and rejection so long that many of them are confused and exhausted. They reflect the challenges that women face in our society at large: the roles we're expected to play, the ideal bodies we're expected to maintain, even the voices we're not expected to have.

Real beauty comes from the inside—from kindness, love, and acceptance.

This sequence, predominantly standing poses, will help build the stability, strength, and courage to stand on your own two feet and to find confidence in the beauty and grace of your body. I include arm balance poses because, as women build upper-body strength, they become more empowered. Recently, a seventy-year-old diva of a woman in my class demonstrated Crow Pose. Everyone was exhilarated and inspired. I asked her afterward what she gets from her yoga practice, and she said with a sly smile, "I love being able to do stuff that people half my age can't do."

Mountain Pose (tadasana). Stand at the front of your mat with your feet together and your arms alongside your body, palms facing inward. Feel the strength of your legs as your feet ground, and draw energy up along your inner legs from your inner arches to the pelvic floor to the light and easy expanse of your chest. Concentrate on balancing your head directly over the center of your chest. Gaze softly over the tip of your nose to a spot on the floor six feet in front of you. Hold for 5 breaths.

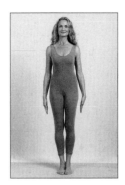

Mountain Pose

Volcano Pose (urdhva hastasana). From Mountain, inhale and reach your arms actively up alongside your ears. Soften your neck and reach your arms higher to lengthen your waist and hollow your belly. Stay in the pose for 5 breaths.

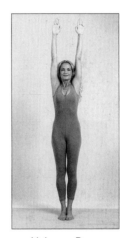

Volcano Pose

Triangle Pose (trikonasana). Stand at the front of your mat and step to the right so that your feet are 3 to 4 feet apart. Inhale as you raise your arms up and out, parallel to the floor. Turn your left foot in 15 degrees and your right foot out 90 degrees. Inhale, lift your chest, then exhale and extend your torso to the right over the plane of your forward leg. Press your right hand on your right shin, a block, or the floor just outside your right foot. Lift your left arm straight up toward the ceiling. As you did in Mountain, root your feet to strengthen your legs and draw energy up from the inner ankles, first to the pelvic floor, then through the top of the sternum. Align your head with your heart center, and turn your upper torso to the left while pushing strongly into your right hand. Stay for 5 breaths. Press down firmly on your left big toe to initiate the lift of your torso, and come to stand on an inhale. Change sides and repeat.

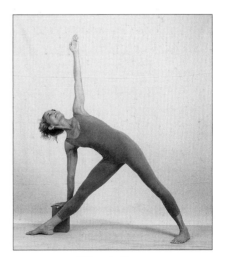

Triangle Pose

Extended Side Angle Pose (utthita parshvakonasana). Turn your left foot in 15 degrees, your right foot out 90 degrees. Exhale and bend your right knee to 90 degrees, knee directly over your heel, thigh parallel to the floor. Exhale and lower your torso toward your front thigh. Press your right hand to the floor outside of your right foot and reach your left arm up and alongside your ear (a). If you can't reach the floor easily, support your hand on a block outside the foot (b) or press your elbow on your thigh (c). Ground the outside of your left foot into the floor. Turn your upper torso to the left and hold for 5 breaths. Press down through your left big toe to come up to stand. Repeat on the other side.

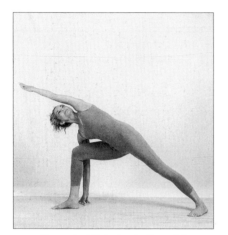

Extended Side Angle Pose (a)

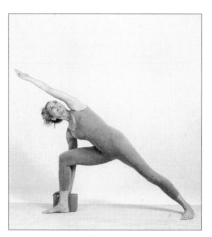

Extended Side Angle Pose
with Block (b)

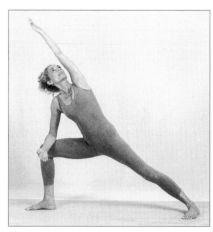

Extended Side Angle Pose,
Arm on Thigh (c)

Half Moon Pose (ardha chandrasana). Come into Triangle Pose to the right. Then bend your right knee and reach your hand to the floor (or onto a block) on the little-toe side of your right foot. As you come into the pose, move the block underneath your right shoulder. Shift your weight forward onto your right leg and right hand. With an inhale, straighten your right leg, making sure it stays externally rotated (so the center of your right knee is aligned over your third toe), and float your left leg up and parallel to the floor. Turn your chest to the left and reach your left arm straight up to the ceiling. Hold for 5 breaths, then bend your right knee and step lightly back to Triangle. Repeat on the left side.

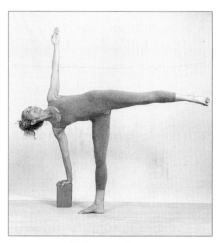

Half Moon Pose

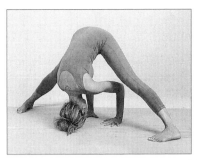

Wide-Legged Standing Forward Bend (a)

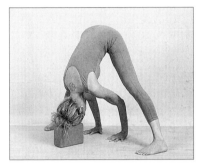

Wide-Legged Standing Forward Bend with Block (b)

Wide-Legged Standing Forward Bend (prasarita padottanasana). Turn your feet parallel to each other and place your hands on your hips. Inhale, lift your chest, and with an exhale, bend forward from your hip joints and come into a forward bend (a). Place your hands on the floor, shoulder distance apart, fingers in line with your toes. Release your head toward the floor. If your head doesn't reach the floor, you can place it on a block (b). Hold the pose for 10 breaths, then inhale, look up, and walk your feet halfway in. Take your thumbs to the top of your buttocks and push them toward the floor to move the torso upright. .

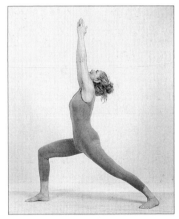

Warrior I

Warrior I (virabhadrasana I). Reach your arms parallel to the floor. Walk your feet as wide as your hands and turn your left foot in 45 degrees and turn your right foot out 90 degrees. Inhale as you raise your arms up and turn your torso to face your right leg. Exhale and bend your right knee toward 90 degrees. Hold for 5 breaths. To come out of the pose, straighten your front leg, turn your feet parallel, and change sides. Repeat on the left side.

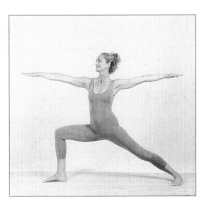

Warrior II

Warrior II (virabhadrasana II). With your legs slightly wider than in Warrior I, turn your left foot in 15 degrees, your right out 90 degrees. Raise your arms parallel to the floor and bend your right knee to 90 degrees. Reach your arms in opposite directions, to broaden and support the lift of the chest. Hold for 5 breaths. To come out of the pose, straighten your front leg and turn your feet parallel. Change sides and repeat on the left.

Wide-Legged Standing Forward Bend (prasarita padot-tanasana). Come into this pose as you did previously, but this time, hook your index and middle fingers around your big toes and press your thumbs into the floor. Straighten your arms, lift your torso, and look forward, lengthening your waist. Maintaining that length, bend your elbows and lower your torso and head into a deep forward bend. Stay for 5 breaths. Inhale, look up, and take your hands to the floor underneath your shoulders. Walk your feet a foot closer together, take your thumbs to the top of your buttocks, and push them toward the floor as you come up to stand. Jump your feet together and stand at the front of your mat.

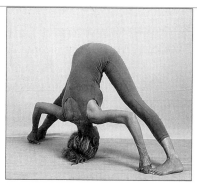

Wide-Legged Standing Forward
Bend Holding Toes

Standing Forward Bend (uttanasana). Inhale and reach your arms straight up to the ceiling, then exhale and swan dive forward from the hips, your legs straight, head hanging. Use your front thigh muscles to actively pull your kneecaps up toward your hips. Hold for 5 breaths, then come up with an inhale.

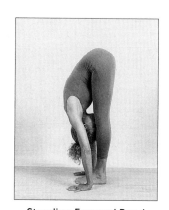

Standing Forward Bend

Chair Pose (utkatasana). From standing, exhale and slowly bend your knees, dropping your thighs toward parallel to the floor. Reach your arms up. Bounce lightly on your legs to root more deeply through your heels. Release your thighs downward and feed your ribs up into the reach of your arms. Hold for 8 breaths, then straighten your legs, release your arms, and stand in Mountain Pose.

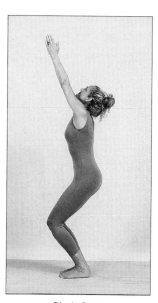

Chair Pose

Eagle Pose (garudasana). Bend your knees and put your right thigh on top of your left, then wrap your right foot behind the left calf (if possible). Press your left elbow into the crook of your right elbow so the backs of your hands face each other. Then pass your left hand in front of your right and bring your palms together (or grab your left wrist with your right hand). Lift your elbows and gaze calmly at your wrists. Stay for 5 breaths, then repeat on the other side with directions reversed. To finish, return to Mountain Pose.

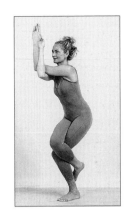

Eagle Pose

Inhale, reach your arms out and up over your head, exhale, and swan dive forward over straight legs into **Standing Forward Bend** (a). Inhale, bend your knees, and look forward, then exhale and step your right foot back to a lunge. On the next exhale, step your left foot back and pull your hips back to **Downward-Facing Dog** (b). Keep your arms straight and continue to pull your hips back. If you feel too much weight on your arms, bend your knees. Hold the pose for 5 breaths. From Downward-Facing Dog, inhale and move forward until your shoulders are over your wrists in **Plank Pose** (c). Reach your heels back. Extend your arms strongly, spreading your chest and looking forward. Keep your abdominal muscles firm but not hard or gripping. Hold for 10 breaths. From Plank, bend your elbows straight back and lower yourself about 2 inches to **Four-Limbed Staff Pose** (d), then straighten your arms back to Plank. If this is too challenging, take your knees to the floor and practice doing push-ups in this position. Repeat 3 times, then pull your hips back to **Downward-Facing Dog** (e).

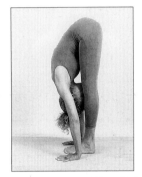

Standing Forward Bend (a)

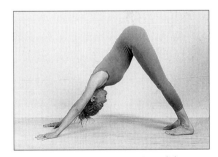

Downward-Facing Dog (b)

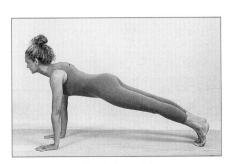

Plank Pose (c)

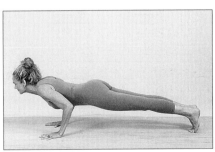

Four-Limbed Staff Pose (d)

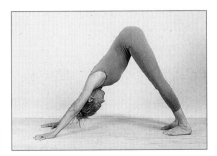

Downward-Facing Dog (e)

Handstand (adho mukha vrikshasana). From Downward-Facing Dog, step your right foot forward one foot. With an exhale, swing your left leg up and push off your right leg (a). Try this a few times. Then step your left foot forward one foot and try on the other side. Go to a wall (make sure there aren't any pictures or knickknacks in your landing area) and try to kick up into Handstand (b). Be sure to keep your arms very strong when you get into Handstand (c). Then come to rest in Standing Forward Bend.

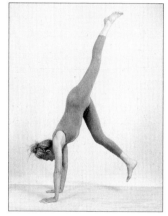

Handstand Kick (a)

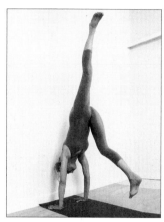

Handstand Kick Against Wall (b)

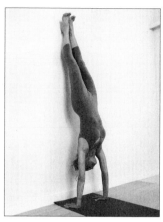

Handstand Against Wall (c)

Child's Pose (balasana). Come to sit with your buttocks on your heels and head on the floor or on a block, palms facing up alongside your hips. Relax your back muscles and feel the weight of your body helping to fold your legs deeply.

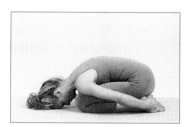

Child's Pose

Crow Pose (bakasana). Push yourself up into a squat with your feet together and your knees wide (a). Let your body hang between your legs. In the squat, work your arms down along your shins, elbows bent, until your inner knees press high onto the outer back arms. Press your hands to the floor, positioning them shoulder distance apart. Shift your weight forward onto your hands and, if possible, lift your feet up off the floor into Crow Pose (b). Pull your heels closer to your buttocks and straighten your arms as much as possible. Lift your head and hold for 5 breaths. Lower your feet lightly back to the floor.

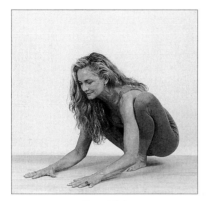
Squat (a)

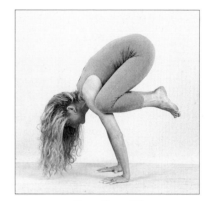
Crow Pose (b)

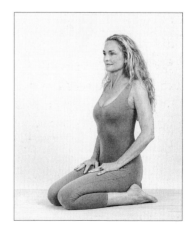
Hero Pose

Hero Pose (virasana). Kneel with your thighs parallel (your knees may or may not be together, depending on the width of your pelvis) and sit back between your feet (have a block handy if your buttocks don't touch the floor comfortably). Close your eyes and dwell in the immense space of your internal universe, realizing the beauty there waiting to be uncovered. Stay in the pose for 20 to 25 breaths, watching your inhalation and exhalation. Focus on what is, nothing else.

Final Relaxation (shavasana). Lie on your back and let your muscles release completely. Empty all expression from your face. Close your eyes. Clean the slate. Stay for 5 minutes.

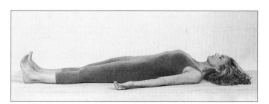
Final Relaxation

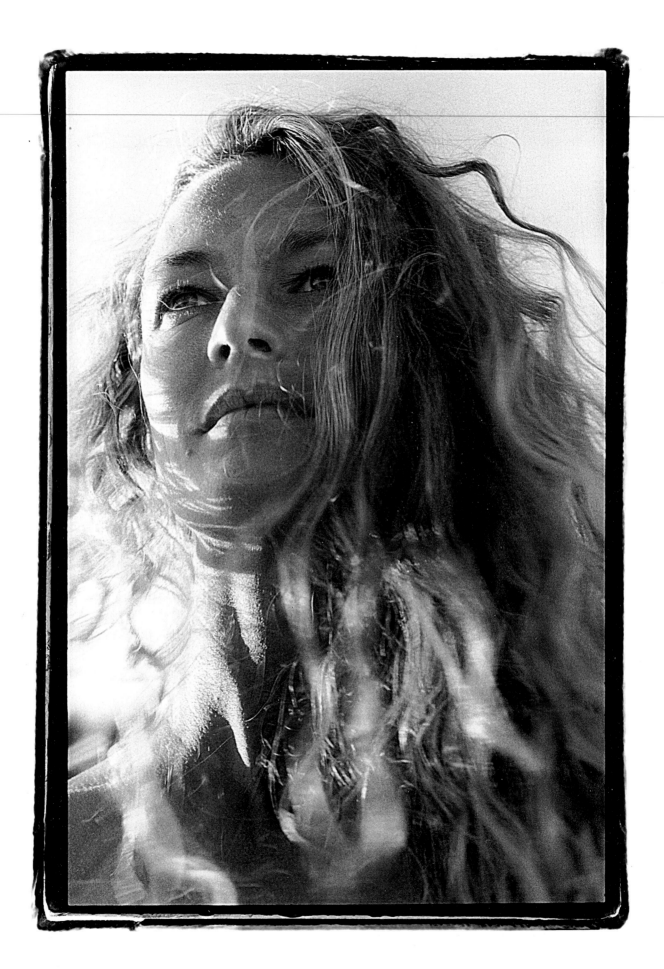

Chapter 6

AWAKENING

There is a cry deeper than all sound
whose serrated edges cut the heart
as we break open to the place inside
which is unbreakable and whole,
while learning to sing.
—"The Unbroken," Rashani Réa

I kept in touch with Robin Saidman after the shoot in Crete, and he continued to book me for occasional jobs. I didn't love working with him; he demanded a lot from me, but he also captured me in photographs like no one else. I was enthralled with his British accent, talent, humor, intelligence, and good looks, so I would find as many reasons as I could to stop by his studio. The first time I realized he was interested, too, was when I happened to be there while he was on the phone making hotel arrangements for a shoot he'd booked me for. He covered the mouthpiece and turned to me. "One room or two?" he asked.

"One," I replied.

Before long I knew I was falling in love with him—but didn't let on.

I spent most of the next few years at Robin's beck and call. We had our own apartments, but by 1988, we were sleeping together most nights. I thought he was the best photographer in the fashion industry. He loved women, which was obvious in his photographs, but he hated playing the game of kissing up to agents and art directors and ended up pissing off most of his clients. He was holding on to his studio by a thread while my career was thriving.

We rented summer houses together for four years on Fire Island and in Brookhaven, Long Island, where his two beautiful children would come from England to spend the summers. In addition to working, Robin and I loved traveling together. We rode motorcycles across Caribbean islands; we rented a Jeep and a tent and embarked on our own makeshift safari in Kenya. We had a blast together.

But Robin wouldn't commit to me. I imagined this was because he was well educated and a brilliant conversationalist, while I was a college dropout and not very cultured. He was also thirteen years older than I was. I thought I was more in love with him than he was with me. Once, when I suspected that his interest was turning elsewhere, I bought us tickets to Jamaica and booked us a nice hotel. We were standing in line to get our boarding passes when Robin turned to me and said, "I can't do this, Colleen. I feel like I'm leading you on." We went back to the city and, believe it or not, continued life as usual. I was so infatuated with him—so in awe of his talent and intelligence—that I never let him know how devastated I was.

One of Robin's fortes was lingerie photography, and I was always jealous of him photographing women in sexy underwear. I became even more insecure, sure that he would eventually leave me for one of those worldly and well-spoken 36-24-36 women.

Desperate to get his undivided attention, I cut my hair short, because Robin talked flatteringly about a model who had short hair. I signed up for night classes at the New School and took courses in current events, art history, and journalism.

Eventually, I got sick of my own insecurity and his ambivalence. I gave Robin an ultimatum: If he didn't propose to me by the following Monday, he could move his things out of my apartment. Monday came and went, and there was no proposal. He pleaded with me and tried to get me to change my mind, but I was firm. Robin moved out.

Emotionally I may have been fragile, but physically, I was in fighting shape. I had been working out with a martial-arts guru named Dwight Wilson. A powerful African American, Dwight was rumored to have trained Israeli commandos. The intense regimens we did with him changed my life. We did standing jumps until we couldn't lift our feet off the floor anymore. We did push-ups until we collapsed. Dwight often said, "If you can learn to kick your own ass, then no one else will be able to." He insisted that we keep going until we were exhausted. Then we would lie on our backs and he would dig his fist into our bellies; if there was any resistance, he would make us get up and continue the workout. If we were completely spent, his fist would virtually touch the floor. At the end of every session, we would lie in puddles of sweat, in what I know now as a deep *shavasana*. When Dwight was satisfied, he would cover us with a towel. Lying on that floor was bliss.

As with final relaxation in yoga, it wasn't unusual for one of us to start sobbing. The emotions held in the body come to the surface. Often this cathartic release is pure sensation without stories attached—old stuff the body has held on to.

Dwight was very selective about who he allowed to work with him. There were about twenty of us and only three women in the group. I did learn to kick my own ass, and, as a result, I kicked a lot of insecurity and fear out of my mind and body. It was the training with Dwight that gave me the courage and strength to leave Robin.

Just days after Robin and I split, I was standing on a street corner in Boston with a model friend named Deirdre McGuire, taking a break from a photo shoot for Saks Fifth Avenue. A black bird literally fell out of the sky and landed at our feet. I turned to Deirdre and said, "Dwight's dead." I don't know how I knew. Later that day I learned that one of Dwight's students had knocked on the door of his bedroom in the studio to tell him that everyone was ready for class. When there was no response, he opened the door and went in. The TV was on and Dwight was sitting upright in his chair, dead. He was fifty-nine years old, and there was no apparent cause of death. I was devastated. Robin was gone, and now I had lost Dwight.

I felt like a needed a break from New York, from modeling, and from my life. It was early summer, and I called my brother Mark. I asked if I could join my brothers on their annual backcountry vacation, which that year was going to be a weeklong canoe trip in Algonquin Provincial Park, a remote area in Ontario, Canada. Algonquin Park has 3,000 square miles of wilderness with 2,400 lakes. The only way to travel around it was by canoe. They had planned a route that involved camping on a different island each night. I assured them I would be able to paddle all day, help portage the canoes, and put up my own tent. They grudgingly agreed and gave me a list of things to bring. I bought the best equipment I could find and packed my journal and my grandmother's rosary.

It was very uncharacteristic of me to "book out" (take time away from my modeling agency), but I knew that I needed to get away, preferably with my family—

rather than calling my answering machine incessantly hoping to hear Robin's voice. The Buddhist nun and teacher Pema Chödrön says that when you are in dire straits, the best thing to do is to go out into nature, lie down on the ground, and look up at the expansive blue sky. It widens our frame and puts things into perspective.

My siblings and I had grown up camping together. Mom and Dad loved being in what they called the "out of doors." Also, it was the only vacation they could afford. We would arrive at a campsite as the sun was going down, pile out of the station wagon, and pitch a huge yellow tent that we all slept in together. I would put on the hand-me-down bathing suit I had inherited from Peggy and we would run to whatever body of water was close by. Dad would put hamburgers and hot dogs on the grill, and my brothers would gather wood for the fire. Once everything was calm, Dad would pull a cold beer out of the cooler and pour Mom a drink. They would both light cigarettes. Their contented sighs said everything—this is what they loved: family and nature.

Today, when I travel with my fancy Samsonite suitcase with its four wheels and multiple compartments, I think back to the little cardboard box I would pack so carefully for the trip. I wonder if I could still need so little to be happy.

The first few days of the canoe trip were strenuous and filled with laughs. I was sore as hell but never let on. Mark's ten-year-old son, Mathew, was obsessed with frogs, and we were constantly catching them and hiding them in each other's tents. The jokes and pranks built through the days. My 6-foot 8-inch brother Ed would emerge from the woods each evening, proudly carrying a small tree under each arm that would keep the campfire going all night.

We were out in the wild with moose, deer, beavers, and bears. Being surrounded by the healing energy of water coupled with working my body and laughing with my family were perfect antidotes for my breakup.

The body relaxes and feels at home in nature. Everyday stress evaporates. You get up with the sun as it dries the nighttime dew and burns through the morning mist. You eat because you're hungry, not because you're bored or stressed. As you sit by the water, your breath seems to match the ebb and flow of the waves lapping against the rocks. I didn't realize how much tension I was holding until I started to unwind. Luckily, there was no time to worry about a British photographer who wasn't in love with me until I was alone in my tent at night.

On our fourth day, the weather was overcast as we set out in our canoes. Farther from civilization now, we saw fewer people on the lakes and portages. That afternoon, we found an island on which to set up camp, but when we discovered other people there, we moved on and found an even more idyllic island nearby.

I always pitched my tent away from my brothers to prove my independence. A few of us went down to the water and were splashing around when Mark appeared. "Get out of the goddamned water!" he yelled, pointing to ominous black clouds on the horizon. It was starting to rain. We jumped out, put on our rain gear, and wolfed down some canned food. As the storm drew closer, we made a fire, and briefly sat around it while John (my youngest brother, an artist) carved a skull and crossbones into a piece of wood. As the rain intensified, we packed up the food, hung it so bears couldn't get it, and scrambled to our tents. For a couple of hours it rained furiously, with intermittent thunder and lightning.

Scared, I wrote in my journal. I put down the book, switched off my flashlight, and lay there, listening to the storm. Suddenly I heard a huge cracking sound and felt something jolt me, hard. My shoulders and heels pushed toward the ground and my hips arched high into the air. Everything went white. My body convulsed with intense pain. Just as suddenly, it was over. I felt profound calm, even though the storm outside was still raging. In that moment, time became elastic and I experienced something close to what I imagine pure contentment (*santosha*) to be. I knew I was dying, and I thought, *I'm in nature, I'm with my family, and I've known love. I'm at peace.*

I must have passed out. The next thing I knew, I was awake. Panicking, I frantically touched my body and realized I wasn't dead. I crawled over to Mark's tent and desperately shook the flap.

"What is it, child?" Mark said, calling me his older-brother term of endearment as he unzipped the flap.

"I've been struck by lightning. I don't want to die alone," I cried. Crawling into the tent, I curled up in the fetal position. As it turned out, Mark's tent had been hit as well. At 6 foot 4 inches, he didn't fit very well and had propped his foot against the metal frame. Later, he said that he felt that he'd suddenly gotten a very severe charley horse in his foot.

We heard yelling coming from Nick and John's tent. John was unconscious, and Nick was trying to revive him. When John came to, he was mumbling that he couldn't feel his legs and thought the water in the tent was his blood. Nick propped him up so he could see his legs. It took a few hours for him to revive fully, and when he did, he was talking gibberish. The zipper from his sleeping bag had burned a long jagged line into his flesh. Save for my nephew, we had all been hit by lightning.

I rode out the rest of the storm in Mark's tent. When the sun came up, John started crying and singing "Here Comes the Sun." We were all frightened and relieved. Saying little, we packed up. As we walked past the flooded fire pit, we saw the piece of wood John had carved the night before; he picked it up and quickly added a lightning bolt above the skull and crossbones.

We paddled hard all day to get to the park exit. I was sick to my stomach from the smell of my own burned hair. At sunset, we pulled into the landing. The park ranger told us that a young German exchange student—one of the group we'd seen the day before at the first island we'd stopped at—had been killed by a lightning strike.

The experience left scars on all of us. John developed a sleep disturbance that lasted for six years. Suffering from cataplexy, he would wake up but couldn't stir his body. Mark suffered bone death in his foot. A few months later, I would suffer my first grand mal seizure, the onset of a disorder I continue to live with.

✦　　✦　　✦

Everyone is "struck by lightning" in different ways at different times. My experience happened to be literal. Besides leaving me feeling extraordinarily lucky to be alive, it zapped me into contemplating *santosha*—"contentment"—which is yoga's second *niyama* or "observance." I had spent most of my life thinking, *I'll be content when I have all A+s.* Or, *I'll be content when Robin proposes to me.* Or, *I'll be content when I have no bags under my eyes.* Or, *I'll be content when I have enough money.* You can wait your whole life and never happen upon contentment. The key is to accept what is and not allow yourself to be jerked between likes and dislikes, attachments and aversions. Accept what is, right now, whether it's comfortable or painful.

I arrived back in New York feeling surprisingly centered and returned to work. A few weeks later, a weather-beaten envelope arrived in the mail. In the upper left-hand corner was a return address: Missionaries of Charity, Calcutta, India. My heart jumped into my throat.

As a child, I had dreamed of becoming a nun. When I was about twelve years old, I'd read a magazine article about Mother Teresa and pored over photographs of her feeding hungry children and saying the rosary in beautiful blue-and-white robes, her face luminous. I wrote her to ask if I could work at her mission in Calcutta. I got no reply—I hadn't really expected one—but I was serious. She had touched me in a lasting way, and over the years I continued to write and ask if I could volunteer.

Now, seventeen years later, I was holding a reply from Sister Priscilla, Mother Teresa's assistant. It said, "You are ready to serve the poorest of the poor. It will be a minimum six-week commitment." I sent back my reply immediately. The only challenge was how quickly I could get my inoculations, finish my modeling commitments, buy a plane ticket, and be on my way.

En route to Calcutta, I stopped to do a one-day job in Los Angeles with a photographer named Peter Lindbergh, whom I admired, for a German cigarette brand. I had been chosen because my body was so buff. They dressed me in an army-green tank top, making me look like a cross between a soldier and a ninja. The stylist asked if I would be willing to have my hair shorn into a crew cut. I was going to India, so I agreed—besides, a crew cut would be a great lice preventive. I was slowly stripping away the strands of my security blanket—Robin, Dwight, modeling, and now my hair.

The day I left, Robin showed up at my apartment with a beautiful notebook. In it, he had written everything I had ever wanted him to say to me—and more. I packed the book in my suitcase and told him that I would think about everything while I was away.

Yoga Sequence:
New Perspectives; Turning Yourself Upside Down

Thinking other people are better than you—whether it's because they are smarter or prettier or more successful—is a form of self-deprecation. It's also a waste of energy. Physically, I probably looked beautiful and healthy enough, but inside, I was a dilapidated house where no music was playing. I cringe when I think about how jealousy turned me ugly. I wasn't practicing yoga's first ethical rule of *ahimsa*, or "nonharming." I was harming myself with desperate attempts to be the woman I thought Robin would love. Getting in touch with my body through Dwight's training saved me. It made me feel kick-ass, strong, and confident. The lightning strike, which was terrifying, woke me up to the preciousness of each moment.

When our world gets turned upside down, we may as well turn ourselves upside down. Poses that are called inversions allow you to see life from a different perspective. Inversions demand presence of mind. You can't be obsessing about your insecurities or worrying about your to-do list when you're in Handstand. Mr. Iyengar said that inversions increase mental function and help to optimize the pineal, pituitary, and thyroid glands. Headstand and Shoulder Stand are known to relieve constipation, too. I use them when I need an attitude adjustment.

This sequence will give you a taste of inversions. Even if you can't balance on your hands or arms, there are many inversion poses that place your head below your heart and create similar benefits. (Potential contraindications for inversions include high blood pressure, glaucoma, menstruation, and pregnancy.)

Supported Downward-Facing Dog (adho mukha shva-nasana). Have a block handy. Fold into Child's Pose (bala-sana), and reach your arms actively forward. Keep your hands and feet where they are, tuck your toes under, and lift your knees off the floor, pulling your hips back until your arms straighten. Then place the block on the floor at one of its three heights (low, middle, high), positioned under your forehead. Support the head in such a way that the ears are aligned between the arms. This is an inversion in which all four of your limbs are on the ground so it doesn't provoke much fear, but it can still be disorientating because you're upside down. Stay in the pose for 10 breaths. Then walk your feet forward and stand at the front of your mat.

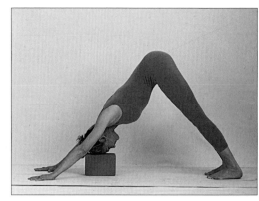

Supported Downward-Facing Dog

Supported Wide-Legged Standing Forward Bend (prasarita padottanasana). Step about 3 feet to the right. Put your hands on your hips, inhale, and lift your chest. Then exhale and fold forward. (If your head doesn't easily touch the floor, put a block or two under your head to support it comfortably.) This is a simple inverted pose most people can do. Mr. Iyengar said it will give you 90 percent of the benefits of Headstand because it stimulates the pineal glands (which produce melatonin, a hormone that affects sleep patterns). The only thing missing will be the keen mental focus that's required in Headstand and other more challenging inverted poses. Keep your legs active and stay in the pose for 10 breaths.

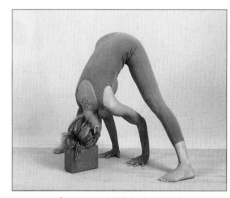

Supported Wide-Legged
Standing Forward Bend

Handstand Preparation (adho mukha vrikshasana). Press your hands against a wall and arrange yourself into as close to a 90-degree angle as possible. Keep your arms and torso parallel to the floor (ears between the arms), legs perpendicular (so the heels are directly below the hips). If your hamstrings are tight, you can move your hands higher. Look at the floor and stay for 5 breaths. Remain here or go into . . .

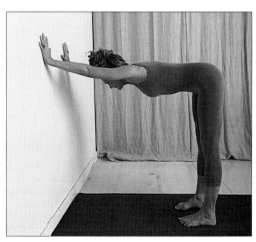

Handstand Preparation

Handstand at the Wall (adho mukha vrikshasana). Approach this pose from Downward-Facing Dog with your hands on the floor at shoulder width, about 4 inches away from the wall. Step your right foot forward, knee bent, and then on an exhale, swing the straight leg high into the air while pushing off the bent leg (a). You may not get all the way up (never say never), but the attempt will focus your mind. This is the safest of the inversions because there's no weight on your neck and head. If you make it into Handstand drive your legs strongly toward the ceiling (b). Stay for 5 breaths. Then come down with an exhale and sit on your heels.

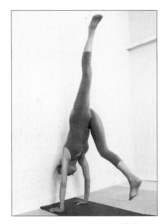 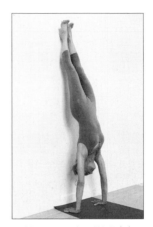

Handstand at Wall (a)   Handstand at Wall (b)

Thunderbolt Pose (vajrasana). Sit on your heels and hold the ends of a block between your palms. Lift it overhead (a), then bend your elbows and slide the block down your back (b). Hold for a few breaths, then raise the block overhead again and lower it toward your lap. Keeping the block between your hands, bring your elbows to touch each other (c) and lift your arms back over your head. Keep your elbows touching as you lift the block as high as you can. Repeat each variation and hold for 5 breaths in each. This will prepare your shoulders for Forearm Stand.

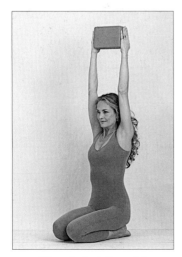 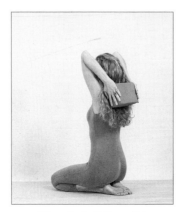 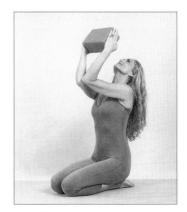

Thunderbolt Pose (a)   Thunderbolt Pose (b)   Thunderbolt Pose (c)

Forearm Stand at the Wall (pincha mayurasana). Place a block at its widest width and lowest height on the floor against the wall. Kneel down and frame the block in the webbing between your thumb and index finger, thumbs pressing on the front side, fingers spreading to either side of the ends, palms down. Lift your hips into **Downward-Facing Dog Variation** (a) and lift one leg at a time into the air, as you simultaneously lift your head and look between your forearms at the floor. Stay for 5 breaths, then try to kick up (b). If you do get up, stay for 10 breaths. This pose is challenging because it requires a backbend and more openness in the shoulder joints.

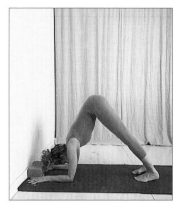

Downward-Facing Dog Variation (a)

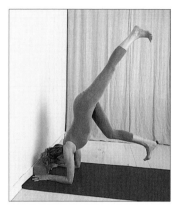

Forearm Stand Kick (b)

Triangle Pose Variation (trikonasana variation). Stand at the front of your mat and step to the right about 3½ feet. Inhale and lift your arms, parallel to the floor. Turn your left foot in 15 degrees and your right foot out 90 degrees. Inhale, then exhale and extend your torso to the right over the plane of the forward leg. Rest your right hand on the floor, on your right shin, or on a block just outside your right foot. Once in the pose, take your left hand behind your head and draw the elbow back to the midline. (This prepares your shoulders for Headstand.) Turn your chest to the left while keeping your legs actively engaged. Triangle Pose requires you to wake up and energize your legs in preparation for inversions. Stay for 5 breaths on each side.

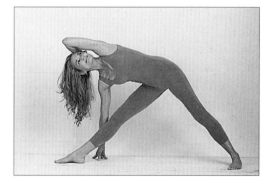

Triangle Pose Variation

Downward-Facing Dog Variation (adho mukha shvanasana variation). Come onto your forearms and knees and interlace your fingers. Press your inner wrists and elbows firmly into the floor (elbows shoulder-width apart) and lift your hips into Downward-Facing Dog Variation. Drop your head and firm your shoulder blades against your back. Press the thighs back strongly, hold for 10 breaths, and then release into Child's Pose.

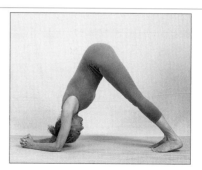

Downward-Facing Dog Variation

Headstand I (shirshasana I) (for the intermediate or advanced student). Interlace your fingers. Press your inner elbows and wrists actively into the floor, then lightly rest the crown of your head on the floor with the back of your head against the bases of your palms. Squeeze your legs together, bend your knees, and bring both heels to the sit bones at the same time—not one at a time, which could strain your neck (a). Then straighten your legs into the air and squeeze them strongly together. Use the strength of your arms and legs to lift weight off your neck and into Headstand (b). It's okay to use the wall to support this pose, but make sure your knuckles are touching it (c, d). If Headstand isn't an option, do a Supported Wide-Legged Standing Forward Bend (see p. 83). Stay in Headstand for 20 breaths if the pose is easy, 10 if not.

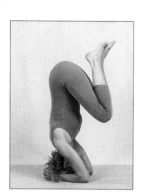

Headstand
Preparation (a)

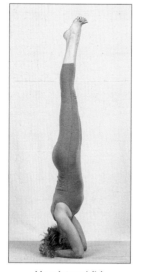

Headstand (b)

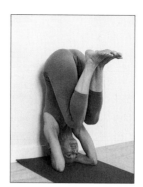

Headstand at Wall
Preparation (c)

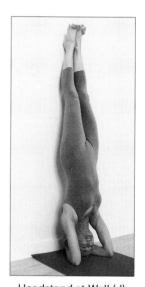

Headstand at Wall (d)

Child's Pose (balasana). Sit on your heels, spread your knees wide, and fold forward, front torso on the thighs, head on the floor for 5 or 10 breaths (a). Then place your chin on a block to reset the natural curve of the neck. Take your arms forward and come up onto the pads of your fingers (b). Stay for 5 or 10 breaths, or for the same length of time that you spent in Headstand.

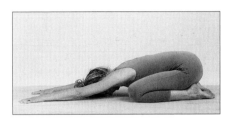

Child's Pose (a)

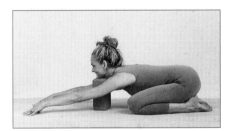

Child's Pose Variation (b)

Supported Bridge Pose with Legs in Air (raised-legs setu bandhasana). Lie on your back with your knees bent and your feet on the floor. Lift your pelvis and place a block at the lowest height so your sacrum rests easily on it. Raise your legs into the air (arms are alongside the body with palms pressing into the floor). If your hamstrings are tight, bend your knees slightly. Stay for 20 breaths. This is an inversion that cools the nervous system from the fire of the other inversions and balances the thyroid and hormones.

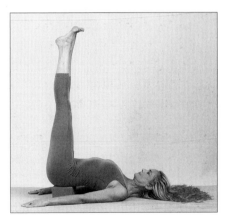

Supported Bridge Pose with Legs in Air

Plow Pose (halasana). Stack 2 or 3 folded blankets and lie with your shoulders on the blankets and your head on the mat (your neck should not touch the blankets or the mat). Swing your legs up and back and over your head and rest your toes on the floor (a) or on a bolster (b) or on a chair (c). Stay for 10 breaths. Slowly roll out of Plow, keeping your head back so it doesn't whiplash forward when the legs and torso touch down. Slide your body back so your shoulders are off the blanket and your pelvis is on the blankets, arms in cactus **(Modified Bridge Pose)** (d). Slide off the blankets and place your hands on your belly; watch 5 cycles of breath. This is another inversion that calms the nervous system and balances the thyroid.

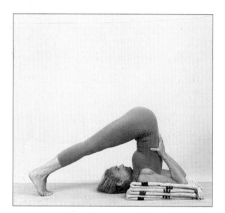
Plow Pose (a)

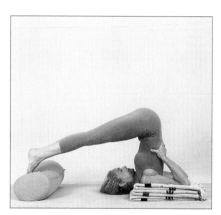
Plow Pose Variation (b)

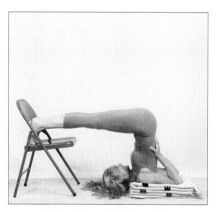
Plow Pose Variation (c)

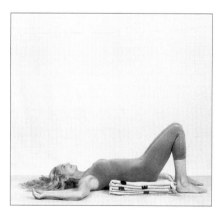
Modified Bridge Pose (d)

Seated Forward Bend (pashchimottanasana). Sit on a folded blanket with legs straight and your torso upright. Fold forward on an exhale (a). You can place your forehead on a bolster if your hamstrings are tight (b). This pose produces an easy exhalation after being out of your comfort zone during inversions and helps the nervous system to relax. Stay for 10 breaths.

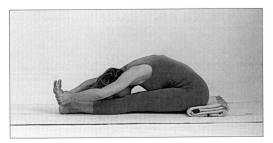

Seated Forward Bend (a)

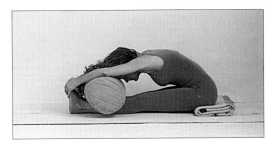

Seated Forward Bend (b)

Final Relaxation (shavasana). Lie down with your arms alongside your body, palms facing up, eyes open or closed. Stay for 5 minutes.

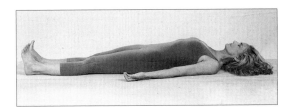

Final Relaxation

Meditation (dhyana). Sit with your legs crossed and focus on the grounding of the tailbone and the opposing action of lifting of the chest. Stay for 5 minutes. All is possible.

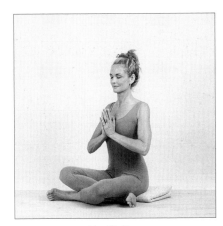

Meditation

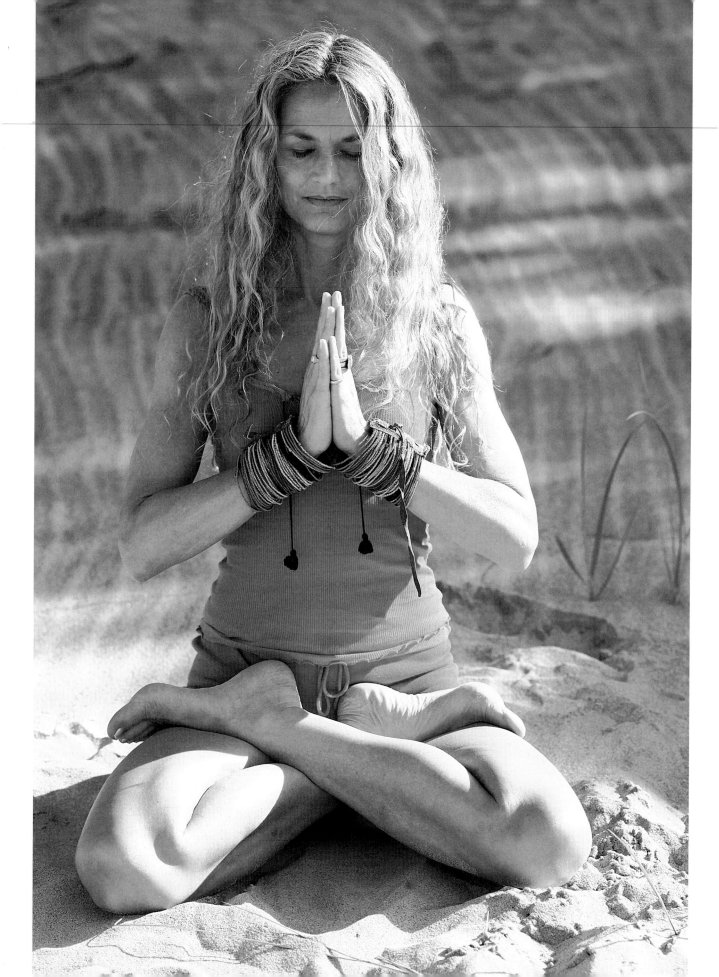

Chapter 7

SERVICE

The fruit of silence is prayer.
The fruit of prayer is faith.
The fruit of faith is love.
The fruit of love is service.
The fruit of service is peace.

—Mother Teresa

My friend and fellow model Dawn Gallagher wanted to go with me to India to work with Mother Teresa's Missionaries of Charity. I'd hoped I would be making a spiritual journey and wanted to do it solo, but Dawn—a 5-foot 9-inch brunette with piercing blue eyes—never took no for an answer. I had no idea if she would be permitted to work without prior approval, but the nuns welcomed her. And she turned out to be the perfect wingwoman. I had committed to eight weeks with the Missionaries of Charity and we decided to leave our return trip open.

Outside the Bombay airport terminal, the scene was chaotic and loud, and the smells in the air were a strange mix of food, burning garbage, body odor, and sweet incense. Stray dogs roamed everywhere, and people, cars, and bicycles spilled over one another.

Everything was strange and confusing, but I immediately felt at home in this crowded, hyperkinetic place. Within seconds beggars set upon us like bees to honey. Locals tried to sell us something (anything), take us somewhere (anywhere), or just ask for money. It seemed to be part of the territory, and not offensive—just a little overwhelming for two jet-lagged New Yorkers. The Indian people seemed to have a sense of relaxation about them. Underneath the craziness, they weren't in a hurry and appeared calm, despite the chaos.

Dawn and I had a week before I was due in Calcutta, and we'd planned to go wherever the wind blew us. A man we met on the plane was on his way to a Siddha Yoga ashram called Gurudev Siddha Peeth, in Ganeshpuri, only ninety minutes from Bombay. He convinced us that the ashram was exactly where we needed to be. I had heard of the spiritual leader of Siddha Yoga, Gurumayi Chidvilasananda, who was stunningly beautiful and loved intensely by her devotees. Siddha Yoga uses the practice of devotion as one of the main vehicles to reach what it calls the "inner divine."

By the time we got to the ashram, I already had "Delhi belly" and was feeling pretty lousy. The girl at the front desk was used to visitors like us showing up with no advance notice and was very accommodating. She took our passports and credit cards and handed us sheets for our beds. When we walked out of the reception area, we came upon quite a scene—something between a holy place and an insane asylum.

In the courtyard, people were sitting around in various blissed-out, trancelike states. A few devotees were quietly chanting, others were meditating, and still others mouthing silent mantras with mala beads in their hands. Clearly, all were on a search for deeper meaning. A few devotees, though, appeared to have lost their minds. One person came up to Dawn and started gesturing in the air around her as if he were pulling something evil out of her body.

The next day, one of the devotees approached me. "Would you like to have an audience with Gurumayi?" she asked. "Sure," I replied. She escorted me to the guru.

Traditionally, a guru (which means "teacher" or "remover of darkness" in Sanskrit) imparts wisdom to students and can serve as a mirror to help them see where they are deceiving themselves. I've met disciples of gurus who have benefitted greatly from the guru-student relationship. In surrendering fully to their guru, they have experienced revelations born from knowing that they were loved unconditionally. A true guru helps remove delusion so there can be an experience of divine love. I've also met gurus who have taken advantage of their students, promising them enlightenment or some kind of "transmission" in exchange for money or sex. The Siddha path is based on the belief that true love is buried deep inside each person and that the guru is there to help bring you to that true self.

Gurumayi was a vision of poise and elegance, and as beautiful as any model, with shiny black hair, perfect teeth, glistening eyes, and adorable dimples. She had a *bindi*, or red dot on her forehead, said to be a symbol of wisdom and spiritual depth. The way she made eye contact with me made me feel as if she had a direct line to my soul. I had stomach cramps and don't remember a word of what she said. Still, being in her presence was moving. The meeting didn't last long, but I felt touched and happy as I hurried back to the hole in the ground that served as a toilet, and then to my dormitory bed.

Later, Dawn came to the dorm and told me that I'd been the talk of lunch; everyone was horrified that I'd worn cutoff shorts and a tee-shirt to meet the guru. Apparently, women were supposed to be covered in her presence. Even though Gurumayi hadn't seemed to notice what I was wearing, I felt terrible. Since I was sick, I stayed another day in my room until I could eat again. Then Dawn and I decided it was time to depart the ashram and took a taxi to Bombay, where we checked into a nice hotel and slept for fourteen hours. Despite some odd moments at the ashram, I was glad we'd gone. We had glimpsed the Siddha message of love and service, and the idea that all of life is an opportunity for freedom and enlightenment made sense to me.

The day after returning to Bombay, Dawn and I flew to Calcutta, which was even crazier than Bombay, with more beggars, lepers, stray dogs, and rickshaw drivers. Intense poverty surrounded us. As in Bombay, many people had an underlying gentleness and a penetrating beauty.

We found our way to the hostel where the Missionaries of Charity volunteers stayed. The courtyard was sweet, with picnic tables and twinkling Christmas lights—a refuge where volunteers would gather at the end of the day to relax and download. Dawn and I settled in to our new home with a sigh of relief.

Early the next morning, we walked with other volunteers to the Mother House. I had the address memorized from the many times I had written to Mother Teresa: 54A Lower Circular Drive. The city was just waking up, and everyone we passed nodded respectfully to us, seeming to know where we were going.

There was one decrepit stoop I walked by every day where a weathered, elderly woman often sat with a girl who looked to be her granddaughter. She would pull lice out of the young girl's hair, making the activity look like a sacred ritual. They both looked tranquil, as if this was their form of prayer. I remember wondering, *How can I get to a place where I feel that kind of peace?* They had so little in the way of material possessions and yet they radiated contentment.

At the Mother House, we met Sister Priscilla, who handed us rosaries blessed by Mother Teresa. She told us about the different "homes" that the Missionaries of Charity operated in Calcutta. There was a home for orphaned boys, a home for lepers, and Kalighat, the Home of the Pure Heart, which was a hospice for the destitute and the dying. The home I picked for my work was Prem Dan, which means "gift of love." It was for adults who were sick, homeless, or mentally unstable. Dawn chose to work at Shishu Bhavan, the Home of the Immaculate Heart, which was for babies whose mothers couldn't take care of them or wanted to give them up for a better life.

Religious affiliation didn't matter. Each person was received as a child of God. People were given last rites according to their faiths—Muslims were read the Quran, Hindus were given water from the Ganges, and Catholics received last rites. Mother Teresa wanted everyone to die with dignity. She said: "A beautiful death is for people who lived like animals to die like angels—loved and wanted."

Every day we would get up and say the rosary with the nuns at five in the morning. The sun shone into the chapel windows, illuminating the selfless women who gave "wholehearted service to the poorest of the poor." Mother Teresa described her call from God "to care for the hungry, the naked, the homeless, the crippled, the blind, the lepers, all those people who feel unwanted, unloved, uncared for throughout society, people that have become a burden and are shunned by everyone." Dressed in white cotton saris with blue trim, the sisters knelt with rosaries in hand, heads bent, reciting the same prayers I had recited under my bedcovers as a little girl. If heroin had been like being wrapped in God's warm blanket, praying in this chapel was like having God's arms wrapped around me.

At Prem Dan, one of my jobs was to help bathe the residents. One man had elephantiasis of the testicles. I think the nuns may have been testing me; as I got used to bathing him, I understood the sacredness of the task. As Mother Teresa used to say, we were bathing God.

Another resident at Prem Dan was Bhalu, which means "bear" in Hindi. I have no idea how old this woman was, but she had been discovered living in a wild place famously inhabited by bears. Bhalu couldn't speak—all she did was grunt. Prem Dan taught me that we don't need to share the same language to communicate. In fact, we don't need to speak at all. Sometimes we communicate more effectively without words. Holding a hand, gesturing, looking into someone's eyes and smiling are powerful forms of expression.

Deep and concentrated observation of the nuns and volunteers who worked at Prem Dan was the best way for me to learn. I wanted to embody their values. As the spiritual leader and teacher Jiddu Krishnamurti wrote, "Observation is action and attention is love." I was attempting to emulate love in action.

No matter how much these people were suffering, they were grateful for our attention. Whether you were changing a bandage, bringing food, or giving an injection, they would always put their hands in prayer position and bow in appreciation. This is the true meaning of *namaste*, which we say at the end of yoga class. It means, "The divine in me bows to the divine in you."

There were times during the day at Prem Dan when I didn't have any specific tasks, so I would do some basic exercises with the residents. I would help them move—lift and lower their arms and legs, even if they were bedridden. Several of them would giggle like children when they saw me coming, and automatically move their arms for exercise as I had instructed. They enjoyed it and seemed to benefit from it. Though I didn't know it, this was my first experience of teaching yoga.

My time at the Missionaries of Charity was a harbinger of things to come. Nearly twenty years later, Rodney and I designed a health and wellness program called Urban Zen Integrative Therapy (UZIT) for patients and caregivers in hospitals. The idea for UZIT started with our friend, the fashion designer Donna Karan. Donna's husband, Stephan Weiss, died of lung cancer in 2001 and had been made more comfortable during his seven-year illness through the modalities of yoga, essential oils, and Reiki. Stephan's wish was to make these techniques more available to hospital patients and their caregivers.

UZIT has now trained hundreds of health-care providers and yoga teachers to use these techniques to help patients feel relief from the common problems that arise during hospital stays. Some of the symptoms we address are pain, anxiety, nausea, insomnia, constipation, exhaustion, sadness, and loneliness.

Occasionally I was asked to work at Kalighat, the home for the dying. It was very intense work, and at first I was afraid. When we volunteers arrived in the morning, we would walk up and down the rows of patients to see if anyone had died during the night. We would carry their bodies into a back courtyard in a manner that was both matter-of-fact and reverent. They had died with dignity and the belief was that they were now with their God. This was Mother Teresa's mission.

Working at Kalighat made death more real for me. When I had worked at Coopers' Rest Home as a teenager, many people died, but I never saw their deaths. I would show up in the morning and Minnie's or Charlie's bed would be empty. It was very unsettling to me, so I would attend their funerals to gain closure. In India, death was in your face on a daily basis.

In yoga studies, we attempt to come to terms with death—of all sorts. Throughout our lives, we are born into new phases and die to others. For instance, we mature from girls to women with the onset of menstruation; we become sexual beings and enter into romantic relationships; we give birth to children, and eventually we release them to the world. Aging (or dying to youth) is a huge challenge in our society; clinging to youth causes a great deal of desperation. If we can learn to loosen our grip a little each day—and be present to what is taking place—we might be happier. If we practice letting go in these smaller deaths, it is said that we'll be better prepared for the big one.

In India, being close to death gave me a more profound appreciation of life. Dying to our egos and selfishness is a daily struggle. That's why, at the end of each yoga class, our last pose is *shavasana*—Corpse Pose.

✦　✦　✦

After working all day in Calcutta, we would make our way back to the hostel. Exhausted, we would sit in the courtyard, drink a few beers, tell stories, and laugh. We felt that we were working purposefully. It felt good to be tired. Peace was the result of giving. Through twelve years of catechism, nine months of college, and a hundred modeling shoots, I hadn't learned this. Now I was seeing and feeling the lesson firsthand.

"What you spend years creating, someone could destroy overnight. Create anyway." This quote by Mother Teresa has become a mantra for me. Beauty lives in the present moment, in the journey, not in the endgame or in the future. I go to her words when I find myself thinking, *What's the use of working so hard? Everything is transitory. My yoga studio won't last. My students will die. I'll die. Why bother to wake up every morning and teach yoga? Why bother loving, when our loved ones will eventually be taken away from us?*

Mother Teresa's quote brings me back to the wisdom and truth that every encounter is sacred: Work anyway. Create anyway. Teach anyway. Love anyway. Buddhist monks spend weeks painstakingly creating intricate mandalas out of colored sand, and then they brush them away and return the sand to the ocean. This traditional ceremony symbolizes the impermanence of life and the world and is a powerful example of "create anyway."

In India, I observed compassion in action. The sisters walked their talk. They weren't lecturing us on how to be caring and kind—they were showing us. The nuns at the Missionaries of Charity bestowed powerful lessons on me without ever saying a word.

Dr. Dianne Connelly, an acupuncturist and spiritual healer, wrote a book called *All Sickness Is Home Sickness*. The title says it all: we have strayed from our homes and it has made us sick. "Home"—that place where we connect to the love, freedom, and contentment that we're all desperately seeking—is buried deep within us. Often, it's the last place we look.

Mother Teresa and the sisters teach that service is the way home. In India, I realized that I didn't need designer boots to be happy. I had two white-and-blue cotton dresses that had cost five dollars each. I wore one on one day and washed the other in a bucket and hung it up to dry. Today, those dresses still hang in my closet next to the designer clothes. They bring me back to a place and time when material things didn't matter—when every day I looked into the eyes of dying human beings and told them they were beautiful.

During several months in Calcutta, I saw Mother Teresa only once, in the chapel. She was saying the rosary with the other nuns. Her head was bowed and her whole body bent from years of prostration to God. She rocked gently as she held her rosary beads with the same hands that had comforted so many dying and unwanted people. My few minutes in the room with her were a gift, but the experience wouldn't have been any less valuable had I never laid eyes on her; she lived within all the nuns and volunteers who worked under her tutelage. She lives in me now, too, and I try to do right by her. She taught that the way to the divine—to peace—is through service.

I had lost my way and slipped and fallen, again and again. After Calcutta, I had even more reason to get back up. I saw a path I could follow. It was time for me to intensify my search for something bigger than a career, a boyfriend—even a family.

Yoga Sequence: Subtle Practices for Difficult Times

How can we transform our yoga practice into service? One way is to bring yoga to people who are elderly, sick, or disabled. Anyone can do yoga, at any age, at any stage of life, and in any place—even bed. Two sequences are included here: One is an in-bed sequence for people who are ill or infirm and one is a chair sequence for caregivers or people who may not be able to stand for the length of a sequence, or who just want a different kind of practice. Rodney and I frequently practice chair yoga. As our friend Donna Karan says: "At one time or another in our lives, we will be the patients and we will be the caregivers." These sequences are for both, but also for people who might just be feeling plain exhausted.

This in-bed sequence articulates every joint and muscle in the body. Even small, seemingly insignificant movements are helpful for the general health of the circulatory, respiratory, and digestive systems—especially for people who are bedridden. They help relieve constipation, depression, anxiety, and insomnia. The person's mental focus is equally important while doing the exercises. If you are leading someone through the poses, watch the person's skin, breath, and facial expressions; if a movement appears uncomfortable, or the person experiences pain or agitation, stop. Endless hours of boredom and isolation can wreak havoc on anyone's spirit. Helping patients do exercises like these can give them some relief in the present—or help them turn the corner toward recovery.

Chair Sequence for Caregivers and Others
(15-Minute Sequence)

This sequence will be beneficial for loved ones or caregivers who sit or stand for long hours and who often neglect caring for themselves. An optimal time to do a chair sequence is when the patient goes for a test or surgery, or is asleep, or for a nurse on a break. It's an all-around sequence that will leave you feeling balanced and provide much-needed relaxation.

Seated Cow and Cat Poses. Sit on the edge of your chair, grab the seat with both hands, and arch your back into seated Cow Pose (a). Then round your back into seated Cat Pose (b). Repeat 5 times.

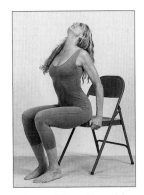 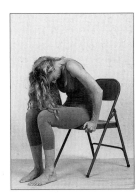

Seated Cow Pose (a)   Seated Cat Pose (b)

Ankle to Knee. Put your left ankle on your right knee; then do the same with the other leg. Stay for 2 cycles of breath each time and repeat 3 times.

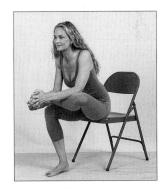

Ankle to Knee

Ankle to Knee Forward Bend. Take your ankle to your knee again and fold forward; hold for 5 breaths. Repeat on the other side.

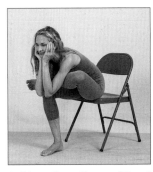

Ankle to Knee Forward Bend

Chair Twist. Sit sideways on the chair with your outer right thigh against the backrest. Hold both sides of the backrest with your hands. Press your feet firmly into the floor as you turn your chest and head to the right. Hold for 3 breaths, slightly untwisting on the inhale and twisting deeper on the exhale. Switch sides. Do this 2 times on each side.

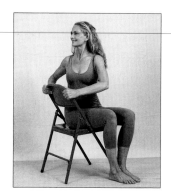

Chair Twist

Sun Salutation with Arms. Sitting on the chair, inhale and stretch your arms out to the side, palms facing up (a). Exhale and press your palms together in front of your chest (b); inhale as you reach your arms up (c); exhale as you drop your arms to your sides (d). Repeat 5 times.

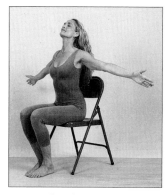

Sun Salutation
Arms Outstretched (a)

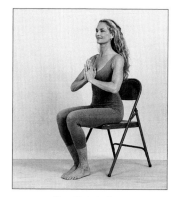

Sun Salutation
Hands to Heart (b)

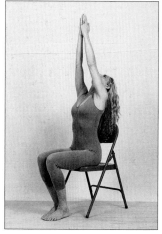

Sun Salutation
Hands Up (c)

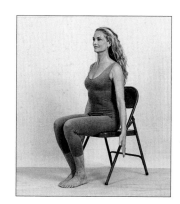

Sun Salutation
Hands at Sides (d)

Chest and Shoulder Openers. Sit near the front edge of the chair, and hold on to the sides of the seat with your hands. Then move your buttocks to the front edge of the seat. Scoot yourself off the seat, then raise (a) and lower yourself (b) as much as you can. As you dip down, keep your elbows as close to shoulder-width as possible. This sequence opens the chest and shoulders and builds the triceps. Repeat 5 times.

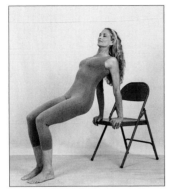

Chest and Shoulder Opener,
Hips Lifted (a)

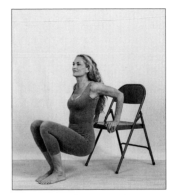

Chest and Shoulder Opener,
Hips Lowered (b)

Upward-Facing and Downward-Facing Dog on Chair. Brace the back of the chair against the wall. Facing the chair, move in to **Upward-Facing Dog** (a) with your hands on the sides of the chair seat. Adjust the distance of your feet from the chair until your shoulders are directly over your wrists. Hold for 3 breaths. Pull your hips back to **Downward-Facing Dog** with your head positioned between your arms (b). Hold for 3 breaths. Keep your hands on the chair and repeat Upward-Facing Dog to Downward-Facing Dog 3 times. Hold the poses for 3 breaths each time.

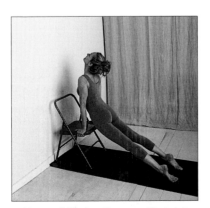

Upward-Facing Dog on Chair (a)

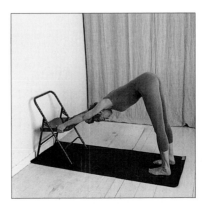

Downward-Facing Dog on Chair (b)

Easy Pose with Forward Bend. Sit on a folded blanket in a cross-legged position facing the chair. Place a blanket on the seat of the chair and rest your head on the blanket with your arms draped over the chair. Change the cross of your legs and repeat, holding for 10 breaths on each side.

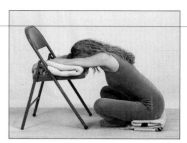

Easy Pose with Forward Bend

Final Relaxation. Lie down on the floor and put your calves up on the chair, with the front edge of the seat pressed into the backs of your knees. Stay for 5 minutes.

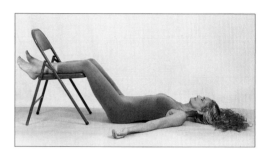

Final Relaxation

In-Bed Sequence
15 minutes

You can practice this sequence yourself. If you are leading someone else through this series, make sure the person is able to see you and ask them to do each movement several times. Try to coordinate their movements with their breath as much as possible.

1. Open your eyes wide and squeeze them closed; repeat 3 times.
2. Turn your head side to side as if you were gesturing no; repeat 3 times.
3. Slowly nod your head yes; repeat 3 times.
4. Stick out your tongue; repeat 3 times.
5. Open and close your mouth; repeat 3 times.
6. Press your head back into the pillow and release; repeat 3 times.
7. Touch your thumb to each finger, one at a time, in order; repeat twice on one hand, then do the other hand.
8. Close your hands into fists, then open them; repeat 3 times.
9. Make circles with your wrists 3 times in each direction.
10. Bend and straighten your arms 3 times.
11. Take your arms alongside your ears, then back alongside your torso 3 times.
12. Reach your right arm across your body and turn your torso and head to the left into a gentle twist. Repeat 3 times on each side.

13. Bend both knees, then drop them to one side. Take 5 breaths, return knees to center, then drop them to the other side and take 5 breaths. Straighten your legs.
14. Press your arms into the bed with elbows bent to get a slight lift to your chest. Repeat 3 times.
15. Bend your knees and step your feet on the bed. Lift your pelvis up about an inch, then lower it down. Repeat 3 times.
16. If possible, roll onto your belly and lie facedown with your forehead on a pillow so you can breathe. Then lift your head 3 times.
17. Take your hands onto the bed and slowly peel your chest up into a baby Cobra 3 times.
18. Lying facedown, lift and lower one leg, then the other. Do 3 times per side and roll over onto your back.
19. Point and flex your feet 5 times.
20. Crunch your toes and spread them 5 times.
21. Make circles with your ankles; repeat 5 times in both directions.
22. "Windshield wipe" your feet to the right and to the left 5 times.
23. Bend one knee and straighten the other at the same time to simulate walking. Repeat 10 times.
24. Bend one knee any amount toward your chest, then straighten it; repeat 5 times per side.
25. Bend your knees and place the soles of your feet together; then lift your knees to step your feet on the bed. The action should look like butterfly wings opening and closing; repeat 5 times.
26. Keeping your knees bent, take your hands behind your head and pull yourself into a small sit-up; repeat 5 times.
27. Roll onto your side with one pillow between your lower legs, one pillow to hug, and one pillow under your head. Rest quietly for 5 minutes.

Rodney and I have seen the value of in-bed and chair sequences thousands of times. On one occasion, Donna Karan, Rodney, and I were visiting the UCLA Medical Center in Los Angeles, which participates in the Urban Zen Integrative Therapy Program. A young girl was in the hospital with leukemia. We did a short in-bed sequence with her, then set her up in a side-lying restorative pose and gave her Reiki with lavender oil on our hands. Then we led her in a short body scan meditation. Afterward, she slept soundly for the first time in six months. We turned to her mother, who hadn't left her daughter's side during her illness. We did a chair sequence with her; after which she lay down on the couch, where we administered Reiki. As we tiptoed out of the room, both mother and daughter were sleeping peacefully. In this work, the practitioner benefits along with the patient or loved one. Service leads to peace, whether it is picking lice from a child's head, feeding the hungry, or giving someone human attention and touch.

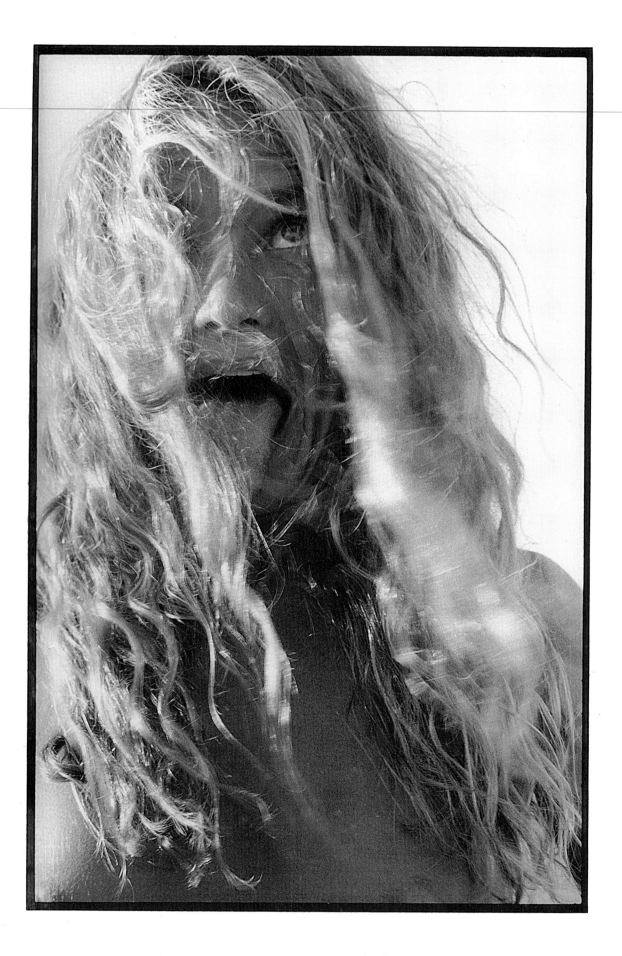

Chapter 8

CHAOS

You are looking outside, and that is what you should most avoid right now.
No one can advise or help you—no one.
There is only one thing you should do. Go into yourself.
                                  —*Letters to a Young Poet*, Rainer Maria Rilke

I arrived back in New York from Calcutta in the winter of 1989. When the taxi pulled up to my loft on West Broadway, I saw a woman in a full-length fur coat getting into a shiny black limousine parked in front of my building, her arms laden with shopping bags from fancy stores. She was screaming at the driver, apparently because he hadn't been waiting for her in the right place. "You idiot!" she shouted. "How dare you leave me standing on the street!" Her face was distorted with rage.

I flashed back to the old woman sitting on the stoop in Calcutta, patiently pulling lice from a child's hair with sheer, unconditional love. The difference between the two scenes was so disturbing it sent me into culture shock. I hurried into my apartment, locked the door, and didn't leave for days.

During the months I had spent with the sisters in India, I had learned that the fruit of silence is prayer, the fruit of prayer is faith, the fruit of faith is love, the fruit of love is service, and the fruit of service is peace. Mother Teresa was rumored to have written these words on the wall of her sleeping chamber. (It was heartening to know that even she would remind herself on a daily basis to go inside to silence.) I'd had a taste of peace; now I knew I needed to find the right form of service.

I admired the sisters for their vows of sacrifice and work for the poor, but I knew I couldn't commit myself in the same ways that they did. I was living in the modern world and wanted a husband, a family, a career, and financial security.

Celibacy wasn't feasible, but was there a middle path I could walk? Could I wear designer boots, have sex, and still serve in a way that would enable peace to prevail in my heart?

In the *Bhagavad Gita*, Krishna tells the warrior Arjuna that "householders"—yogis who choose to live in the world and have families—can attain the same enlightenment as renunciates. Swami Vivekananda writes, "It is useless to say that the man who lives out of the world is a greater man than he who lives in the world; it is much more difficult to live in the world." My own family had nourished me, sacrificed for me, and protected me. I was ready to find the person with whom I could create my own family.

A few weeks after I'd arrived in Calcutta, I had written two letters. One was to Robin, telling him that, although I appreciated his change of heart, I didn't want to be with him because I felt that I would never find my voice as his partner. I wrote a second letter to a man who was in love with me and who, even though we had never formally dated, would be a loving, caring husband. I told him I would marry him. I put stamps on the letters and dropped them in a mailbox on the street. Unfortunately, I never got the memo about the Indian postal system. If you put letters with stamps in a mailbox, the stamps will be stolen and the letters thrown away. Neither of my letters reached their intended recipients. When I got home, the friend I had agreed to marry was happily engaged to someone else. Robin had bought me a ring.

Robin asked me out and took me to an elegant Indian restaurant—appropriately called Nirvana—overlooking Central Park. As we sat down, I could tell he was nervous. He clumsily pulled a box out of his sports jacket, cleared his throat, and knelt down on one knee. "Colleen, will you marry me?" he asked in a sarcastic British formal voice. But I knew he was serious.

"Yes," I answered.

The truth was, I was still in love with Robin. I had imagined this moment for years. During shoots, when another photographer would ask me to exude happiness, I would imagine Robin asking me to marry him. My infatuation was stronger than my reservations, and I did a 180. I still had a lot to learn about myself; my relationship with Robin would prove to be a fertile learning ground.

Our wedding took place in my loft four months after I returned from India, with the reception at Robin's photography studio. I wore a white, micromini Giorgio di Sant'Angelo dress. It was a raucous night; unbeknownst to us, someone was passing around marijuana joints laced with angel dust, and most of the wedding guests were high as kites. The wedding photographer must have been high, too, because in the photographs that came back, many of the guests' heads and feet were cut off. My brothers were in heaven, watching beautiful models in tight, short dresses dancing to reggae music. When the band played Bob Marley's song "Three Little Birds," its lyrics "Don't worry 'bout a thing, 'cause every little thing's gonna be all right" perfectly captured my reality at that moment.

Music is the language my family speaks, and song lyrics are my inspiration. As a young girl, I would pore over Bob Dylan's album sleeves for hours, memorizing every lyric as if it had been written specifically for me. Each stage of my life relates to music. Carole King's *Tapestry* album carried me through adolescence. Dylan taught me tender love with songs like "Lay, Lady, Lay" and "Tonight I'll Be Staying Here with You." Melissa Etheridge empowered me, and I felt like Annie Lennox met me at my lowest points by writing "Oh God." Jason Isbell's three-word refrain "know you're enough" from his song "Cover Me Up," should be embedded in every woman's brain. The rawness and honesty of Fiona Apple breaks me open and helped inspire this book.

My life had changed. I was married. I had a thriving career and was back in the family fold. I was living my dream, but something was missing. I felt less natural in this seemingly perfect existence than I had felt in chaotic India. I realized that service needed to be part of my life, even though the form it would take hadn't yet been revealed.

In 1987, the year before I'd gone to Calcutta, I'd taken my first yoga class. At the time, I was still running and boxing and taking whatever aerobic boot camp classes I could fit into my schedule. My friend and next-door neighbor Kathy Law (now Kathy Freston) was into yoga, and kept pestering me to try it. I considered myself an athlete, so I pooh-poohed her, but eventually I agreed. The class was on Broadway in SoHo with a teacher named Nancy Vinik. I followed along the best that I could, listening attentively to every word she said. There was a lot I couldn't do, which surprised me. I considered myself in great shape, but I didn't have balance or flexibility. As people moved into Fish Pose (a backbend) I thought, "Wait a minute, my spine doesn't do that." I was both humbled and intrigued.

After class, I went out onto Broadway, a street I'd walked down hundreds of times before, but this was different. The lights, the colors, and the smells of the city seemed crystal clear. It was as if I had been wearing blinders and someone had re-moved them. Kathy and I walked quietly and mindfully home, as if on a pilgrimage. The yoga door had opened, even if it would be a while before I walked through it wholeheartedly.

Around that time, *New York* magazine had hired me for a photo shoot that re-quired me to look like I knew how to box, so they paid for me to take a few lessons at Gleason's Gym in Brooklyn. The second I walked in the door, I was in love with the whole environment—the smell of sweat and leather, the guys yelling at each other, and their fists hitting the bag with a grunt. I admired the intensity and dis-cipline of the boxers and their trainers. It was a guru-disciple relationship. When they were in the ring, they were fully present, and their minds were focused.

The first time I walked into Gleason's I think everyone thought I had wandered in by mistake. Bruce Silverglade, a boxing promoter, invited me into his office and we formed an immediate connection. He told me the dos and don'ts of being a woman in the gym. The miniskirt I was wearing was a "don't."

Many of the old ex-boxers like Jake LaMotta were usually hanging around. Being raised in a half-Italian family with five brothers had prepared me perfectly for this environment. I felt right at home. The place was grungy, the perfect coun-terpoint to life as a fashion model. I ended up being a regular at Gleason's, working with trainers Hector Roca and Barry Funches, who had coached champions such as Larry Holmes, Mike Tyson, George Foreman, and Muhammad Ali.

I was among the first female boxers at Gleason's. After a while, more women started coming to the gym—mainly police officers—so I had women to spar with. One of my bouts was against a woman named Sparkle Lee. The fight got a lot of media attention because it took place the same week that my cover for *Cosmopoli-tan*'s Beauty Guide hit the stands. Fortunately, I was much taller than most of the girls, so getting hit in the face wasn't much of a danger. But Sparkle, who was a cop, did break a few of my ribs during our fight. That was pretty much the end of my boxing career. Years later, Hector would take on another woman training for a role—Hilary Swank for *Million Dollar Baby*.

Just as I thought I was hitting my stride, life was about to catapult me into a se-ries of crises. Robin and I weren't planning a child yet, and I was on the pill. When I missed my period, I decided to take a home pregnancy test. The moment the plus sign appeared, I went into shock. What would I do about work? The day I found out, I was on the subway and burst into tears. A woman sitting next to me leaned over. "Are you all right?" she asked.

"I'm fine," I gulped, between sobs. "I'm pregnant!"

Trying to be helpful, she gestured to a Planned Parenthood advertisement in the subway car.

"No," I said. "I want this baby."

The poor woman looked as confused as I felt.

My mom, the devout Catholic, was a fervent right-to-life activist. I, on the other hand, was equally fervent in my belief that women have a right to choose, even though I would never have been able to bring myself to have an abortion. So I made peace with the fact that I was pregnant. Robin and I found out the baby was a boy, and we named him after my troubadour hero, Dylan. I continued to work and felt so normal that there were days I had to remind myself that I was actually pregnant. I later learned that the reason I wasn't having usual pregnancy symptoms was that my progesterone level was extremely low. I miscarried in my second trimester. It was a devastating loss.

A couple of months after the miscarriage, I was in Los Angeles for a month-long modeling job for Avon Fashions. Every evening I went to a step aerobics class at the gym next door to the hotel. One night, after jumping over one too many steps, I ended up on the floor in agonizing back pain. I was carried out of the gym and back to my room at the hotel, where I called 911. A doctor came and gave me injections of muscle relaxants and steroids.

Amazingly, I still managed to finish my commitment with the Avon Fashion Catalogue. I modeled those terry cloth robes as if they were silk and cashmere, and as though I felt like a million bucks. I took more pain pills, had to be carried off the set, and flew home to New York, where I lay horizontal, in excruciating pain for the next few months.

A famous back doctor I went to see told me my pain was psychological—probably resulting from financial worries, he posited. This was laughable considering I would earn in the mid-six figures that year. He prescribed more pain pills and suggested I consider psychotherapy.

Robin and I drove home to see my parents for Thanksgiving—rather, Robin drove with me lying on the backseat of the car, floating dreamily on Percocet. My mom and dad totally freaked out when they saw me and made an appointment with a doctor in Fort Wayne, who prescribed an MRI. After reading the results, he said I needed emergency surgery for a ruptured disk that had lodged in my sciatic nerve.

As soon as I got back to New York, I got a second opinion from Dr. Robert Snow, who concurred. Dr. Snow said that my spine looked like I had jumped off the Empire State Building and landed on my feet. Three days later, I underwent a type of back surgery called a diskectomy. Dr. Snow removed the disk and left the connecting vertebrae to fuse on their own. In the hospital, the self-controlled morphine drip gave me that old familiar drug bliss. Part of me wanted to keep pressing the button for more, but instead, I asked for the pump to be taken away. Intuitively I knew there was a better way to deal with pain and craving.

Was back surgery a blessing? Maybe. Because of the surgery, I was forced to give up impact sports like step aerobics and running. I had dabbled in yoga during the eight years since I'd taken that first class; now I was ready to move into its full embrace. Once we tune in and listen, the body becomes increasingly difficult to ignore. I had paid a high price for not listening to mine. I resolved to stop beating it up and to fall in love with it instead. Not only would yoga fulfill my exercise requirements—in time, it would inspire and instruct me in every realm of my life: physical, emotional, psychological, spiritual, ethical, and yes, even sexual. I have been monogamous to yoga ever since.

Yoga Sequence: Honing Our Attention

Becoming rigid in a chaotic situation is like being caught in a riptide and struggling against it. If you fight, you'll get exhausted and be swept away. Yoga is like a life raft that teaches us to observe and listen and allow ourselves to be carried by the tide until we find a place where we can safely break its hold.

Yoga is a muscle; the more you practice, the easier and more natural it becomes to create space to witness your internal turmoil. To hone attention, our initial step is focusing on alignment in the poses. In yoga we examine both the gross and the subtle bodies: the "gross" body is the physical; the "subtle" body consists of the mind and the energetic forces that flow through us. It's usually easier to understand how to move your thighbone back and lift your chest than to find inner space through meditation. *Asana* prepares our bodies for the more subtle practices such as *pranayama* (breath work), *dharana* (concentration), and *dhyana* (meditation).

Eventually, we may be able to sit with all that arises, observing sensations that may include rage, fear, jealousy, and anger. If you can sit and watch these emotions rise and fall, observing that they ebb and flow like everything in nature, you can release their constricting hold over you. There will be times when your asana practice will call up these emotions; in these moments, you may realize that your inner world does not have to be a battleground. A strong asana practice burns impurities and releases tension in the body. As the practice calms the ripples of the mind, we see glimpses of peace. Especially in times of upheaval, you can count on your yoga practice to be a bridge from chaos to calm.

During asana practice, our minds become sharper and more attentive. This sequence is a wake-up call, like speaking sharply to a child to get his or her attention. It's also a strength sequence; we go back and forth between poses that require strength in the legs, the arms, then in both the legs and arms. Adding elements of gaze and breath creates focus to keep the mind from wandering.

Our yogic gaze—keeping the eyes softly focused—is a constant throughout a sequence. Being aware of your breath and how it moves and is absorbed in the body is an even more subtle meditation. *Pranayama* demands a sharp and undistracted mind, which brings us to the doorway of formal seated meditation. There's no "you" and "I" when we practice this kind of attention. There's no goal or desire, just intense listening and responding. It's our work on attention—like this strong fifteen-minute sequence—that can help us center ourselves in times of chaos.

Plank Pose. Come to your hands and knees, tuck your toes under, and straighten your legs as you move your shoulders over your wrists, arms perpendicular to the floor. Reach back strongly through your heels and engage your abdominal muscles, broadening your upper chest and upper back. Plank is a demanding pose that builds strength and focus. Look across the room with soft eyes and hold for 5 breaths. Then walk your feet between your hands.

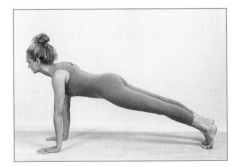

Plank Pose

Chair Pose (utkatasana). Bend your knees and lower your thighs toward parallel to the floor. Raise your arms and "sharpen" your elbows. Gaze over the tip of your nose to a spot about six feet in front of you. Hold for 8 breaths. Exhale and fold forward over bent knees.

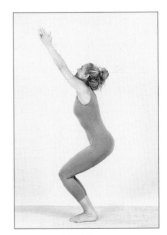

Chair Pose

Downward-Facing Dog (adho mukha shvanasana). Place your hands alongside your feet and walk back to Downward-Facing Dog. Press your legs strongly back; relax your neck and head and gaze softly at your legs. Hold for 5 breaths.

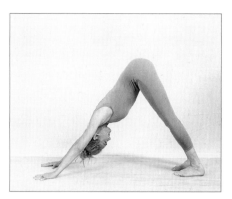

Downward-Facing Dog

Warrior II (virabhadrasana II). Step your right foot forward between your hands, ground your back heel as you turn your toes in 15 degrees, and windmill your arms up and out so they are parallel to the floor. Open your chest and hips to the left. Let the reach of your arms help spread your chest. Press strongly through your left heel, and bend your right knee toward 90 degrees in line with the center of your foot. Gaze out over your right hand. Hold for 8 breaths, then exhale and bring your hands to the floor on either side of your front foot and step back to Downward-Facing Dog. Repeat with the left foot forward.

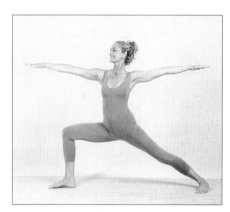

Warrior II

Side Plank (vasishthasana). From Downward-Facing Dog, shift onto the outside edge of your right foot and stack the left leg on the right in Side Plank. Then shift your weight onto your right arm and turn sideways, swinging the left arm straight up to the ceiling (a) into Side Plank. Lift your hips as high as you can, and gaze up at the top hand. If the full pose is too difficult, modify by resting the bottom knee on the floor (b). Hold for 3 breaths on each side; finish in Downward-Facing Dog.

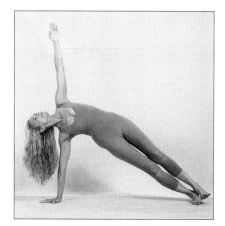

Side Plank (a)

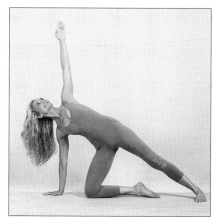

Side Plank Variation (b)

Warrior I (virabhadrasana I). Step your right foot forward between your hands, ground your back heel, and turn your toes in 45 degrees. Reach your arms alongside your ears. Bend your front knee toward 90 degrees. Lift your chest with the reach of your arms, and gaze at your thumbs. Take your hands to the floor and step back to Downward-Facing Dog. Repeat with the left leg forward, finishing in Downward-Facing Dog.

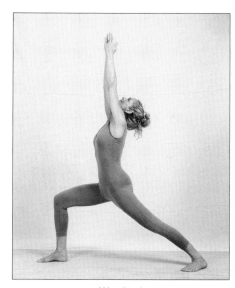

Warrior I

Handstand (adho mukha vrikshasana). Place the short end of your mat at a wall and take Downward-Facing Dog with your hands 4 inches away from the wall. Walk forward about a foot, and on an exhalation swing one leg straight up behind you (a). Propelled by a kick from your bent-knee standing leg, launch yourself toward or into Handstand (b). Try to coordinate the movement of the legs on an exhale and be sure to keep the arms strong. Gaze between your thumbs. Do 5 hops per side, then rest in **Child's Pose** (c) for 5 breaths before sitting in **Staff Pose** (d).

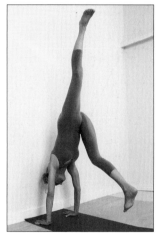

Handstand Kick at Wall (a)

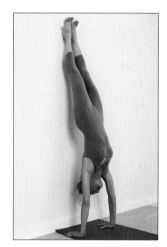

Handstand (b)

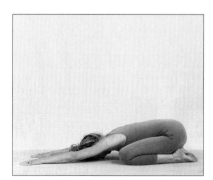

Child's Pose (c)

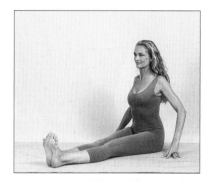

Staff Pose (d)

Reverse Tabletop (purvottanasana). Place your hands six inches behind you, fingers pointing forward, then bend your knees to plant your feet about a foot in front of your sit bones and lift your hips. Try to bring your torso and thighs as parallel to the floor as possible. Drop your head back, but if that feels strained, keep it in a neutral position. Hold for 3 breaths. Keep your gaze over the tip of your nose. Repeat, but this time, if possible, walk your legs straight to **Inclined Plane** (b) and press your soles to the floor. Hold another 3 breaths, then lower down with an exhale and sit in Staff Pose.

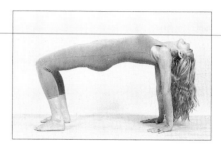

Reverse Tabletop (a)

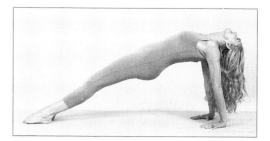

Inclined Plane (b)

Boat Pose (navasana). Place your hands behind you and on the exhale, lift your legs diagonal to the floor so that your body forms a "V." Reach your arms alongside your legs, pumping them a few times (a). If this is too difficult, bend your knees and stay on the front of your sit bones (b). Another option is to keep your hands on the floor (c). Gaze softly at your feet and lower your legs with an exhale.

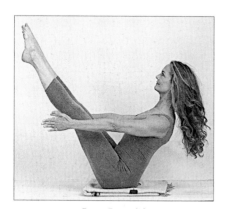

Boat Pose (a)

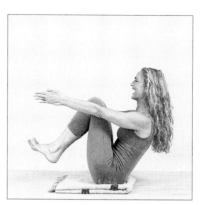

Boat Pose with Bent Knees (b)

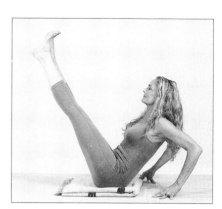

Boat Pose Variation (c)

Reclining Easy Pose (supta sukhasana). Lie down on your back. Cross your left shin in front of your right, then inhale to raise your arms over your head. Bend your right elbow and slide your hand behind your head and down toward your left shoulder blade. Then take your left arm and slide it down your back toward your right shoulder blade, creating a pillow for your head. Switch arms by putting the other arm on top and switch legs by putting the right shin in front of the left. With the eyes closed, drop the gaze below the cheekbones. Hold for 20 breaths.

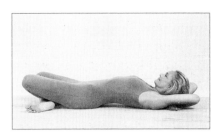

Reclining Easy Pose

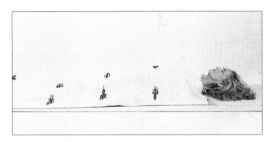

Final Relaxation with Blanket

Final Relaxation (shavasana). Lie down on your back and cover yourself with a blanket. Feel the containment, warmth, and comfort of the blanket. Keep your mind focused on the sensations of the body. Stay for 5 minutes.

Meditation (dhyana). Sit cross-legged in a comfortable position with your eyes softly open, seat raised, and knees supported as necessary. Your tether is your focus on your breath and gaze; sit in the eye of the storm and observe the whirlwind for 3 minutes.

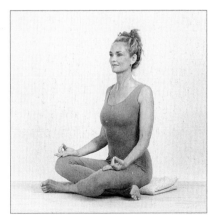

Open-Eyed Meditation

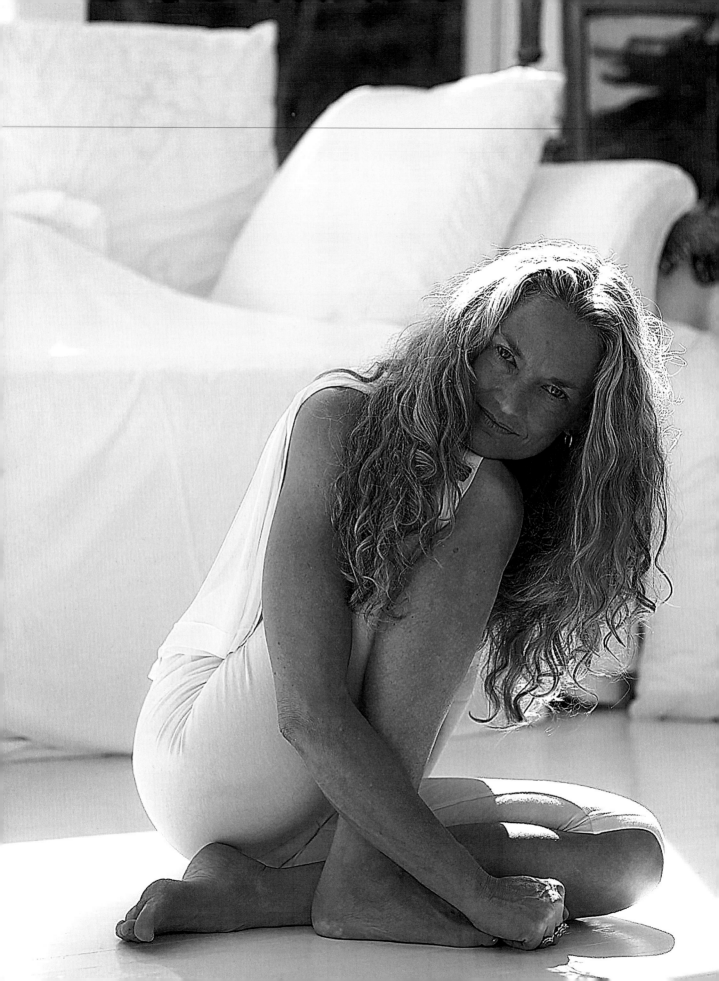

Chapter 9

FEAR

So first of all, let me assert my firm belief
that the only thing we have to fear is fear itself—
nameless, unreasoning, unjustified terror
which paralyzes needed efforts to convert retreat into advance.
—Franklin Delano Roosevelt

When I encountered epilepsy I got to know fear from a whole new perspective. As a seizure is coming on—just before the convulsions start—I have an intense feeling of déjà vu called an aura. It's kind of a cool feeling, almost like an awakening. Everything goes into super-slow motion. Time loses its linear quality. I have a feeling that the moment has happened before, or I've dreamed it. I'm old and young at the same time. Sometimes I'm able to talk as it starts, enough to tell Rodney or whoever is around what is happening. Real fear is waking up after the seizure and not knowing your name, or how old you are, or where you are, or what happened to you. Fear is not recognizing your daughter or your spouse sitting next to you or seeing the look of angst in their eyes as I slowly piece my world back together again. Fear is not knowing if I will regain my mind.

I was first diagnosed with epilepsy in 1989 when I was thirty years old. I never know when a seizure will occur, or how severe it will be. There isn't a single trigger I've been able to figure out. Zen monks often clap their hands loudly and say, "This could be it!"—meaning, you could die this instant. I don't need that kind of reminder. It's always with me.

For years, I have lived in fear of seizures, of the embarrassment of having one in public, of getting badly hurt, even of dying. I'm now trying to be grateful for my seizures and the lessons they have taught me. I've had more than one hundred of them since my late twenties, and they have been among the most brutal, but important teachers in my life.

◆ ◆ ◆

I experienced my first grand mal seizure in India, though I didn't understand what was happening to me at the time. Dawn Gallagher and I had finished our service with Mother Teresa's Missionaries of Charity, and we decided to travel from Calcutta to Varanasi to see the *ghats*, the descending broad stone terraces that lead down to the River Ganges. Varanasi is where dead bodies are brought to be cremated, and where spectacular rituals of fire worship to the Lord Krishna are conducted on huge, burning pyres. Dawn and I boarded the train in Calcutta along with hundreds of people, chickens, and goats. We paid for an upgrade so that we could have seats in a cabin for the twelve-hour trip.

I hadn't been feeling well in general, and on the train I began to feel worse. Dawn had been so careful about not drinking the water or eating food from the street. She was equally meticulous about taking her malaria medicine. But, thinking I was invincible, I hadn't taken the same precautions. She continually pestered me about taking my malaria pills, but I thought the whole notion was ridiculous. I had read that there were many strains of malaria, and the medicine protects you from only a couple of them. Plus, the malaria pills made me feel lousy. When we boarded the train my head was pounding, my stomach was flip-flopping, and I was confused. Six hours later, I started moaning. Dawn tried to ask people how much farther it was to Varanasi. But nobody spoke English.

All of a sudden I started to shake harder and harder. I was foaming at the mouth, my eyes were rolling back in my head, and my body was convulsing. Finally, a man who happened to be a doctor and spoke English came to our aid. When the seizure subsided, he checked my pulse—it had plummeted to twenty-five beats per minute.

"She's really, really sick," the doctor said to Dawn.

"We have to get off the train at the next stop," Dawn said.

"Madam, you can't get off," he said. "We're in the middle of nowhere. You'll have to wait for Varanasi, which is six hours away."

"I don't know whether she'll make it," Dawn replied, panicked.

"I don't know whether she'll make it either," he said.

For the next six hours, I was mostly unconscious. Dawn held my hand and sobbed and prayed. When we pulled into the Varanasi station, she frantically rounded up some men to help take me to a nearby hotel—our friend on the train had told us in no uncertain terms not to go to a local hospital. He gave Dawn the name of a private doctor to call. We got to the room and while we were waiting for the doctor, I went into another convulsion and fell off the bed.

The doctor arrived, looked at me, and said, "I must start administering medicine through an IV right away." Dawn objected. "I need to know what you're giving her and if the needle is clean!" The doctor said, "Madam, if I don't start now, she will be dead in fifteen minutes."

When I woke up, I was confused and frightened. I was in a strange room, hooked up to an IV. My entire body was in excruciating pain, and I could hear the hotel manager asking Dawn for an address where my body might be shipped, if necessary.

The convulsions had broken several of my ribs. I had also bitten my tongue and chewed up the inside of my mouth pretty badly. My head was pounding and I felt like I had been run over by a Mack truck. Eventually things quieted down, and when the doctor arrived on the second day, Dawn took the opportunity to take a much-needed shower. I was going to make it.

Forty-eight hours later, I was strong enough to leave the hotel and told Dawn I still wanted to see the burning *ghats*. She tried to dissuade me, to no avail, so we ventured down to the Ganges. The scene was incredible; corpses were being carried by the dozens down the stairs and thrown onto enormous fires. The smell of burning flesh was intense. There were dead bodies floating in the river, some of which were babies. According to Hindu tradition, corpses are cremated or destroyed by fire, which returns the body to the earth and frees the spirit for its ongoing journey.

Saddhus, the divine, holy (and sometimes seemingly crazy) Hindu mystics, were practicing austerities on the riverbanks; one man had been holding his arm in the air for years, and it had withered to skin and bone. Others were standing for long periods on one leg. Many wore loincloths, or less, and their bodies were painted and their hair had never seen a comb or barber. They were practicing an extreme form of *bhakti* (devotional) yoga through *tapas*, in which austerities are considered an offering or sacrifice that can burn up the impurities and ignorance of this life, which will merit a better reincarnation. The scene was colorful and wild, and like so much of the complexity in India, it also somehow felt completely normal to me.

When Dawn and I were ready to make our way back to Calcutta, we decided to fly (enough of trains). When we got to the Varanasi airport, who did we see sitting in the lounge but the doctor who had treated me at the hotel. As far as I was concerned, he was the man who had saved my life. Dawn, however, became agitated and starting yelling at him, calling him a pervert, and demanding our money back. I was stunned. Dawn then told me that when she had come out of the shower in the hotel room, she had found the doctor touching me in inappropriate ways. He clearly didn't want Dawn to create a scene, so he quickly peeled off some bills, shoved them at Dawn, and walked away. We flew back to Calcutta, said our good-byes, and headed home.

◆　◆　◆

After our return to New York, I continued to think that the seizure was a crazy fluke due to something I had picked up in India (the doctor had suggested I might have contracted cerebral malaria). But two months later, it happened again. I had been called for jury duty and was sitting on a hard, dark brown bench in the Lower Manhattan courthouse, answering questions to determine whether I would qualify for a particular case. The next thing I knew, I opened my eyes and a nun was standing over me, holding my hand and telling me that I was beautiful and that God loved me. Was I in heaven? If so, it was a very hectic and noisy place. I had no idea what had happened. I should have been petrified, but this nun was stroking my hand and telling me that I was loved.

I was in the emergency room of Saint Vincent's Hospital, in the West Village of New York City, and I'd had a grand mal seizure. I had been brought by ambulance to the hospital. I had been unconscious for four hours. As with the first seizure, when I came to, I thought, *What am I doing here? Why are my body and head throbbing? Why am I nauseated, and why is there blood on my shirt? Why am I hooked up to beeping machines?*

The blood was from biting a bit of my tongue off. The pain was a result of the intense contraction of every muscle in my body and the nausea was probably from shaking so violently. Robin came to get me, and we immediately scheduled an appointment with a neurologist, who did a barrage of tests and explained that I had epilepsy, a neurologic and central nervous system disorder. Grand mal seizures result from an unexplained electrical discharge in the neurons of the brain. My symptoms were classic: violent convulsions, loss of consciousness, biting of the tongue, spasming limbs, arching of the back, foaming of the mouth, and rolling of the eyes.

No one really knows what causes epilepsy. For me, it could have been a result of the brain injury I suffered from the car crash at age fifteen, or possibly malaria, or drug abuse, or being struck by lightning. It could have been all, none, or a combination of the above.

As a result of seizures over the years, I've suffered concussions, broken bones, bruises, and numerous bloody mouths, but one of the toughest challenges has been dealing with the shame and embarrassment, and the fear of not knowing when a seizure will strike. At my weakest (and most Catholic) moments, I wondered if I'd done something wrong and was being punished. I felt like damaged goods, a freak. I wanted to curl up in the safety of home and let life pass me by. I felt that I was traumatizing those close to me who had to witness it and who lived with me in fear of the next one. I do understand that my shame and embarrassment are partly the result of how our culture views disorders such as seizures. Interestingly, other cultures, like the Balinese, view seizures as energetic awakenings, which are a gift.

✦   ✦   ✦

In 2013, because I hadn't had a seizure in several years, I decided, unbeknownst to my doctor, to wean myself off my medication. It was a bad call. I started having mild auras, then stronger ones. I didn't tell anyone because I didn't want to go back on the meds and thought that, with my advanced *pranayama* and meditation, I could control the seizures. One day in May, when I had been off my medication for four months, Rodney and I were in the shower when I had a grand mal seizure. Rodney had to push my body against the wall because there wasn't enough time for him to get me out of the shower. It was hellacious for him to have to pin me there while I seized, but the alternative was to chance having me crack my head on the marble tub. As a result of that seizure, I suffered several compres-

sion fractures in my spine. The medications I'd quit taking had made the seizures less frequent and, when they did happen, less severe. But I'm stubborn, and
told myself that the seizure in the shower was a fluke. I refused to go back on my
medicine.

Three months later, I was giving a talk to a group of potential teacher trainees
at Yoga Shanti when I had another major seizure and fractured my tailbone and
one of my thoracic vertebrae. After that, I made an appointment with a neurologist, who ordered an MRI and an EEG. The scans showed the brain injury I'd
suffered as a teenager at the stem of my brain. He couldn't connect the injury to
epilepsy, but he told me that I needed to go back on medication, and he put me on
Lamictal.

For nearly thirty years I've tried every alternative antiseizure remedy, from acupuncture to hypnotism to homeopathy to biofeedback to taking fistfuls of supple-
ments, but the seizures recurred. After the seizure at Yoga Shanti I was willing to
follow my doctor's advice. He also recommended a ketogenic diet, a high-fat, low-
carbohydrate regimen that was developed in the 1920s to treat pediatric epilepsy.
I've done my best with it and believe it's part of the solution.

The biggest transformation has been my acceptance. When I take my little
white tablets every day, I'm grateful for Western medicine. I supplement it with
diet, acupuncture, and yoga—but I don't feel defeated anymore. Instead, I feel
awakened to the fact that I'm not in control of everything. Maybe we're born into
bodies that challenge us to learn lessons we haven't yet understood. All situations,
no matter how painful, can be opportunities for growth.

I know I'm not invincible. I don't drive a car or swim alone anymore. When I
went back to India three years ago, I took my malaria medicine, drank only bottled
water, and didn't eat food sold on the street. I know we're lucky to have the bodies we have, no matter what they bring with them. Still, it's easy to make excuses or
create stories when you're afraid of being hurt or embarrassed.

One week after my 2013 seizure, I was invited to teach yoga to 4,500 people at the Grand Palais in Paris. I thought about declining. But what was I going
to do—sit at home and stop everything? I flew to Paris with my dear friend and
fellow yogi Kari Harendorf. I stood on the stage with my broken vertebrae and
chewed-up tongue and faced my terror of having a grand mal seizure in front of
thousands of people (actually millions, because it was live-streamed). I've commit-

ted to keeping an open mind to any and all solutions, but I won't let fear control or diminish my life.

Mr. Iyengar must have sensed this during a workshop Rodney and I took in Colorado. When it came time for Headstand, I told him that I no longer did them because I have epilepsy, and several times after long Headstands, I'd felt like I might go into seizure. He told me to get into Headstand. I obeyed. When the rest of the class came down, he told me to stay up. When he finally told me to come down, I did, and immediately started to join the class, which had moved into Hero Pose. At this point, he slapped me lightly and said, "*This* is your problem. It is not Headstand. You do not let anything absorb. You are moving too fast from one pose to the next. Perhaps you do this in your life as well. Slow down. Stay in Child's Pose for as long as you were in Headstand."

He was right—I do move too fast from one thing to the next. That lesson from Mr. Iyengar continues to remind me to let the absorption of the present moment sink in. I continue to practice Headstand, but I always stay in Child's Pose for as long as I was in Headstand. I take this lesson off the mat, too, and notice when I'm rushing mindlessly from one thing to another.

July 2014 would have marked a seizure-free year. But in June, as eighty students were lying in *shavasana* after a class at Yoga Shanti Sag Harbor, I turned off the music and reached for a poem by Maya Angelou I was going to read. Just then, the familiar feeling of déjà vu started in my belly and rose to my throat. I stayed standing, thinking that I could wait out the aura. I felt my feet. I breathed calmly. Then I realized I couldn't talk. The last thing I remember was Yoga Shanti's manager, Lisa Olsen, peeking around the corner to see if everything was all right. When I woke up, a man I vaguely recognized was asking me questions I couldn't answer. All I could do was cry. I fell back asleep, and when I woke again he was still there.

"What is your name?" he asked.

I was blank.

"What is your daughter's name?"

Again, nothing.

Then he asked, "What's your father's name?"

"Nick," I replied.

The man was Rodney and he didn't try to hide his tears of relief. I was coming back.

It took me five days to feel like my brain synapses were firing properly. I wrote an email to the eighty students explaining my seizure disorder and apologizing for busting their yoga buzz. I still live with fear about when the next seizure will come. I accept that any moment may be my last and celebrate every month that is seizure-free. Each day I get up, put on my yoga clothes, roll out my mat, and plan a sequence for class. I fall in love with yoga and the perspective it provides me—all over again.

Yoga Sequence: Facing What Scares Us

There's no guarantee of safe passage in life. Pema Chödrön teaches the importance of not running away from difficult emotions, that if we can sit quietly with them, eventually the expanse of blue sky will appear. This teaching is helpful when fear starts to paralyze me or propel me into frenetic retreat, and over the years I have found the following Buddhist meditation useful.

It goes something like this: Sit down and notice where you hold fear in your body. Notice where it feels hard, and sit with it. In the middle of hardness is anger; sit with the anger. Go to the center of anger and you'll usually come to sadness. Stay with the sadness until it turns to vulnerability. Keep sitting with what comes up; the deeper you dig, the more tender you become. Raw fear can open into the wide expanse of genuineness, compassion, gratitude, and acceptance in the present moment. A tender heart appears naturally when you are able to stay present. From your heart, you can see the true pigment of the sky. You can see the vibrant yellow of a sunflower and the deep blue of your daughter's eyes. A tender heart doesn't block out rain clouds, or tears, or dying sunflowers. Allow beauty and sadness to touch you. This is love, not fear.

Mr. Iyengar believed that backbends help us face our fear—of death and of the unknown. This sequence culminates in backbends, which demand both fearlessness and vulnerability. Backbends open the door to the heart; they are life affirming. We elicit fear in yoga so that we can walk courageously through it.

Mr. Iyengar also said that you master fear by mastering backbends; they pierce the protective shell we think keeps us safe and makes us face the unknown behind the illusion. This sequence is designed to gradually soften hardness or resistance that results from fear. We build up to it. Open your heart and embrace the day for its beauty. Hear the birds chirp, feel the air on your skin, listen to music. Hold your loved one's hand—all with awareness of impermanence.

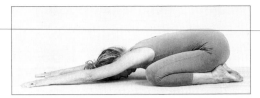

Child's Pose (balasana). Sit on your heels, big toes touching, with knees spread wide. Lay your torso in between your legs, rest your forehead on the floor, and reach your arms overhead on the floor. This pose promotes a sense of safety because all your internal organs are protected.

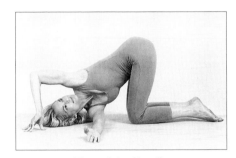

Child's Pose

Thread the Needle. Lift up onto your hands and knees. "Thread" your right arm under your left and rest your right outer shoulder and cheek on the floor. Press your left fingertips onto the floor to help navigate the twist. Stay for 5 breaths, then change sides and repeat. This pose spreads your back muscles and prepares you for the upcoming backbends. Lie on your belly and make a pillow for your head with your hands. Let the spine settle. Stay for 5 breaths, rocking gently from side to side. Notice how the spine moves with the breath.

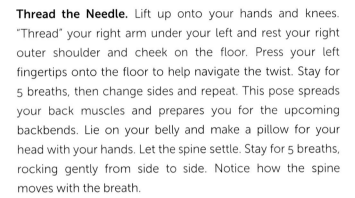

Thread the Needle

Still on your belly, lengthen your legs away from your pelvis, press your bent elbows to the floor, and rest your chin in your cupped hands in **TV-Watching Pose (niralambasana variation)** (a). Slide your elbows forward to open your shoulders. Gaze softly over the tip of your nose to a point on the floor several feet in front of you. Stay for 8 breaths. This is the first of several backbends and takes place from the safety of the belly on the ground. You are beginning to open your heart without exposing vulnerable organs.

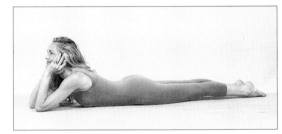

TV-Watching Pose (a)

Press your forearms on the floor, parallel to each other, with the elbows positioned directly under your shoulders (so the upper arms are perpendicular to the floor). With an inhale, press your palms against the floor and pull your chest forward with your arms into **Sphinx Pose (supported salamba bhujangasana)** (b). Lift your chin and your chest as if they were tethered together. Press your feet into the floor as you reach your legs long; they are the foundation for all backbends and protect the lower back from strain and overuse. Stay for 5 breaths, then lower back to the floor.

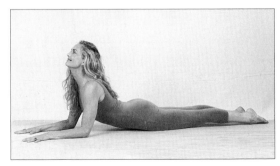

Sphinx Pose (b)

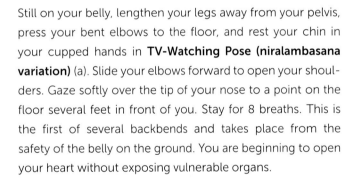

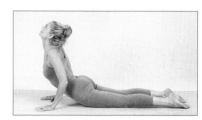

Now slide your hands back alongside your chest. Press your palms into the floor and pull your chest forward and up into a bent-arm **Cobra Pose (bhujangasana)** (c). Stay for 3 breaths, then lower down. Inhale and draw your chest forward and up as you slowly straighten your elbows as much as possible without straining your back (d). Stay for 3 breaths, then lower down.

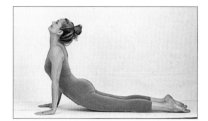

Cobra Pose (c)

Cobra Pose with Straight Elbows (d)

Rest your arms on the floor alongside your torso, palms up. Press the backs of your hands and the tops of your feet into the floor and draw your chest forward and up. Stay for 3 breaths (e). Lower down for a few breaths, then inhale and repeat. Straighten your arms overhead and lift your arms, head, and legs off the floor into **Locust Pose (shalabhasana)** (e,f). Hold for 5 breaths.

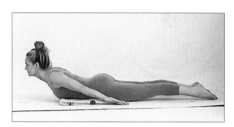

Locust Pose, Variation (e)

Now position your hands on the floor alongside your chest and press the tops of your feet against the floor. As you straighten your elbows, pull your chest through the arms and fire up your legs to lift off the floor into **Upward-Facing Dog (urdhva mukha shvanasana)** (g). Stay for 3 breaths, then lower down and repeat the sequence.

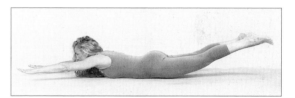

Locust Pose (f)

Stand on your knees, grab the sides of your mat, and press back into **Downward-Facing Dog** (h). This variation opens your shoulders for the upcoming backbends. Stay for 8 breaths.

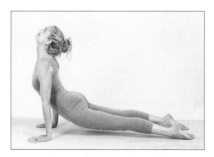

Upward-Facing Dog (g)

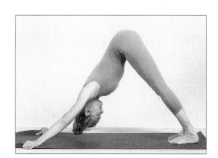

Downward-Facing Dog (h)

Hero Pose (virasana). Widen your feet and sit between them on the floor or on a block. Interlace your fingers behind your head and drop your head back into your hands as you lift your chest toward the ceiling for 5 breaths (a). Change the interlace of your fingers and repeat. Place your hands or forearms behind you on the floor and lean back to open the fronts of your thighs and shoulders (b) in preparation for Upward Bow (urdhva dhanurasana). Then, if possible, lower all the way down to the floor into **Reclined Hero (supta virasana)** (c) or onto a bolster (d). Stay for 5 breaths, then come to your hands and knees and push back to Downward-Facing Dog, pedaling your feet as necessary to stretch the calves and hamstrings for 5 breaths. Walk to the front of your mat.

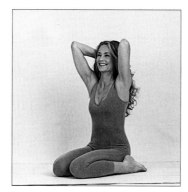

Hero Pose, Hands Behind Head (a)

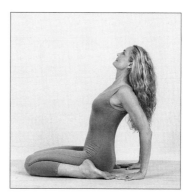

Reclined Hero Pose Transition (b)

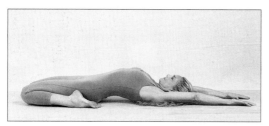

Reclined Hero Pose (c)

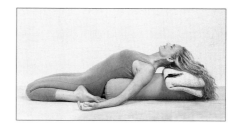

Modified Reclined Hero Pose (d)

Bend your knees, bring your thighs as close to parallel to the floor as you can, and reach your arms vigorously up into **Chair Pose (utkatasana)** (a). This prepares your legs to ground down as you lift into Upward Bow. Stay for 3 breaths. Inhale and stand in **Mountain Pose** (b). Hook your thumbs into your front armpits and feel your chest and head being lifted by an invisible hand inside your sternum in **Modified Standing Drop Back** (c). As you drive your legs back, press your hands into your sternum and lift into them, leaning into a backbend. Reach your arms out to the sides, palms facing up, and lift your chest a little more into **Standing Drop Back** (d). Stay for 5 breaths in each stage. Inhale, bend your knees into **Chair Pose** (e), then exhale and fold forward without straightening your legs. Step your right foot back to a lunge, take the right knee to the floor, and reach your arms alongside your ears, arching up and over your back leg into **Crescent Moon Pose (anjanasana)** (f). Take your hands to the floor and step forward into **Chair Pose** (g). This pose is an excellent preparation for backbends since it opens the front spine, shoulders, and hip flexors. Finish by stepping back to **Downward-Facing Dog** (h). Repeat sequence on the other side.

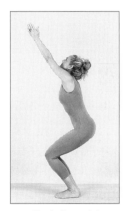
Chair Pose (a)

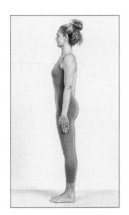
Mountain Pose (b)

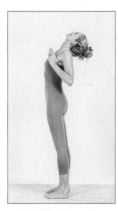
Modified Standing Drop Back (c)

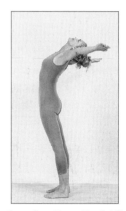
Standing Drop Back (d)

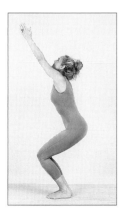
Chair Pose (e)

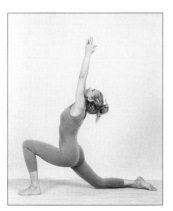
Crescent Moon Pose (f)

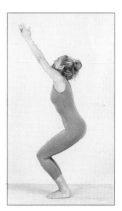
Chair Pose (g)

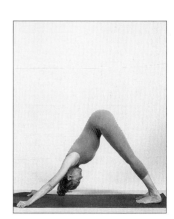
Downward-Facing Dog (h)

Warrior I (virabhadrasana I). From Downward-Facing Dog, lift your right leg into the air and step your right foot forward between your hands. Ground your left heel, lift your torso upright, and reach your arms alongside your ears, arching your chest up and over your back leg. Bend your front knee toward 90 degrees and hold for 3 breaths. Step back to Downward-Facing Dog and repeat on the other side. Warrior I teaches us to strengthen the legs and ground the heels, essential for pushing up into Upward Bow Pose. It also stretches your front spine and opens your shoulders in preparation for backbends. From Downward-Facing Dog, walk forward, and move through Chair Pose to Mountain Pose.

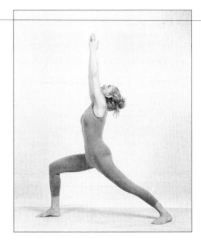

Warrior I

Lord of the Dance Pose (natarajasana). Bend your right knee, bring the heel to the buttock, and grab your right ankle with your right hand (a). Draw your thigh back. Reach your left arm up and touch your thumb and index finger together. Hinge forward over the standing leg and lift your back leg higher (b). Repeat on the left side. This pose will stretch the hip flexors. Return to Mountain Pose, take Chair Pose, and walk back to Downward-Facing Dog.

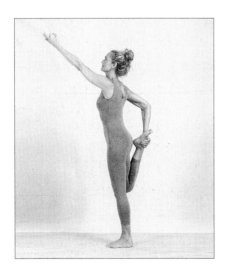

Lord of the Dance Pose Prep (a)

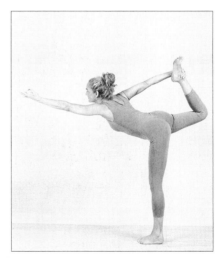

Lord of the Dance Pose (b)

Camel Pose (ushtrasana). Kneel on your mat or on a folded blanket. Lift your head and chest into a backbend, first with your hands on your hips (a), then with your fingers interlaced behind your head (b), and then with your hands on your inner back thighs (c). If possible, take the full **Camel Pose**: hands on heels or pointed toes (d). Hold for 3 breath cycles per variation, then come to all fours, cross your shins, sit down behind your feet, and lie on your back, arms alongside the body.

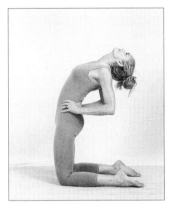

Camel Pose Preparation (a)

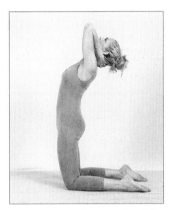

Camel Pose Preparation (b)

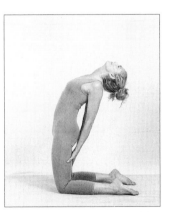

Camel Pose Preparation (c)

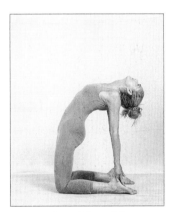

Camel Pose (d)

Fish Pose (matsyasana). Straighten your legs and press them strongly together and down. Push your elbows into the floor to lift your chest and place the crown of your head on the floor. Hold for 3 breaths and repeat.

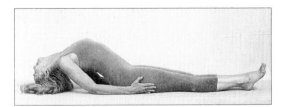

Fish Pose

Upward Bow (urdhva dhanurasana, optional). Lie on your back, bend your knees, and step your heels close to your buttocks. Press your hands to the floor beside your head, elbows bent, fingers pointing toward your shoulders (a). Inhale and lift your pelvis off the floor, then press up onto the crown of your head, making sure not to put too much pressure on the head and neck (b). From the power of your legs, lift your hips and straighten your arms, as much as possible, into **Upward Bow** (c), a perfect pose for facing the unknown—and your fears. Stay for 5 breaths, then lower down, lie on your back, and extend your legs.

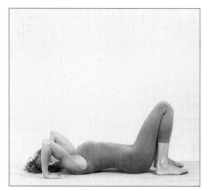

Upward Bow Preparation (a)

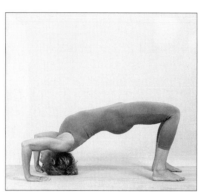

Upward Bow Preparation (b)

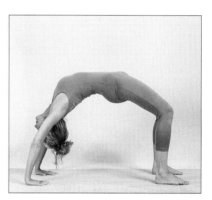

Upward Bow (c)

Reclining Big Toe Pose (supta padangushthasana). Place a strap around the ball of your right foot and straighten your leg to the ceiling. Press your straight left leg strongly into the floor. Stay for 8 breaths. Change sides and repeat. After the backbends, this pose brings the spine back to neutral and stretches the hamstrings, which tend to tighten in back-bends. Neutralizing the spine is very important for the safety of the disks before moving into any other category of poses.

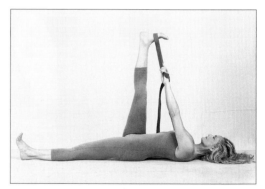

Reclining Big Toe Pose

Reclining Bound Angle (supta baddha konasana). Bring the soles of your feet together with your knees open to the sides and evenly supported with rolled-up blankets or blocks so you don't feel a stretch in the inner thighs (a). Stay for 10 breaths. Next, keep the soles of the feet together and place them on a block at the lowest height or on a rolled-up blanket for 8 breaths (b). Most backbends require internal rotation of the thighbones in the hip sockets, so this pose rebalances the hips with external rotation.

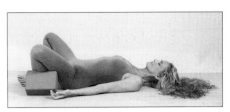

Reclining Bound Angle Pose with Blocks (a)

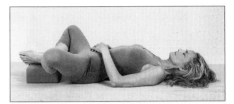

Reclining Bound Angle Pose
with Blocks Variation (b)

Final Relaxation (shavasana). Lie down on your back; place a bolster under your knees and the small roll of a blanket under your neck. Stay in shavasana for 5 minutes.

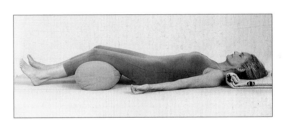

Final Relaxation

Meditation (dhyana). With quiet awareness, dig to the center of any hardness you feel until you perceive the expanse of blue sky. Sit with what is until the tenderness of a genuine open heart is revealed.

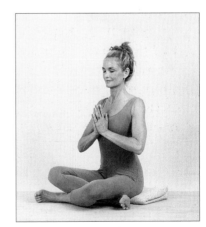

Meditation

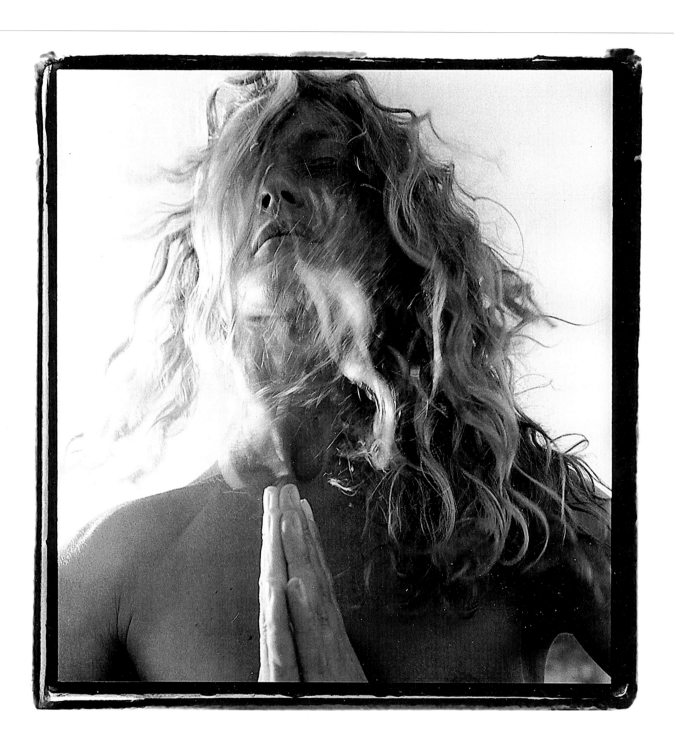

Chapter 10

EXPECTATION

My happiness grows in direct proportion to my acceptance,
and in inverse proportion to my expectations.
—Michael J. Fox

My miscarriage had left me heartbroken. Afterward, I realized that I wanted to be a mother more than anything in the world, and I became obsessed with the idea of having a baby. I would take my temperature, check my mucus, read my horoscope, consult psychics, pray to Mother Mary, and demand sex from Robin, especially when the stars seemed to be aligned. But I was so uptight that for the first time in my life, sex wasn't fun and the pregnancy kit became a stressful ritual. No wonder I wasn't conceiving. I would lock the bathroom door and have a moment of nervous excitement thinking, *Maybe this is it.* When the minus sign appeared, my heart sank.

One week after my back surgery, Robin and I flew to Nevis for a short vacation. We had a lovely, relaxed time, and voilà, conception!

When we got back, I took the test and knew in my bones that the plus sign would appear. I was right and I immediately fell in love with being pregnant. I've never felt as sexy and radiant as I did during the next nine months. After all the years of counting calories as a model there was something liberating about watching my waistline expand and my belly grow. The final modeling job I did during my pregnancy was when I was twenty weeks. I'd been hired to do a campaign for Hugs tee-shirts, and we were shooting a series of posters that were going to hang in every Kmart in America. Even though I was sucking in my stomach, there was no disguising it—my belly was round, my face was full, and, for the first time in my life, I had breasts.

I'd always been self-conscious and critical of my modeling photographs, and the only photo that I've ever liked unequivocally—the only one in which I think I look truly beautiful—was one Robin took of me when I was seven-and-a-half months pregnant. He photographed me topless, wearing cutoff jean shorts; my hair was wild and I had a joyful, sexy twinkle in my eye. To this day, I keep that photograph in my office. When I gave birth, I weighed 170 pounds, 45 pounds over my regular weight. I didn't regret one of those pounds.

I now belonged to a special club that I hadn't known existed. Women started smiling at me and striking up conversations. They gave me advice and shared their own stories of pregnancy. I felt loved and accepted by other women, which wasn't the case before. I was nauseated throughout my pregnancy but happily so. When I was fifteen weeks along, I was on a modeling job and woke up feeling completely fine. It was such a dramatic change that I called an ambulance and went to the hospital because I was nervous that I felt so good. A nurse reassured me by showing me the baby's healthy heartbeat.

During those nine months, my sex drive was in overdrive. I felt like a voluptuous goddess. Sex had always been a deeply satisfying pleasure for me—just as my mother said it should be. But this was the first time I felt fully like a woman.

I've never been shy about talking about sex to our kids (or to anyone else). When my daughter Rachel was turning thirteen, I said to her, "Honey, shall we have 'the talk'?" She rolled her eyes. "Mom! You've been having 'the talk' with me since I was two years old!" When Rachel was a junior in high school, I told her that masturbation was the best remedy for PMS. She put a pillow over her head and shrieked, "Am I hearing my mother encouraging her daughter to masturbate?"

My fantasy while I was pregnant with Rachel was to have a pure, natural birth in a warm pool in my living room with candlelight, incense, and music. Because of the miscarriage I'd suffered, my pregnancy was considered high-risk, so my doctor advised me to give birth in a hospital. I was disappointed and turned that disappointment on myself. I felt like a failure for not fulfilling my expectation of this birth.

I was determined to make my hospital birth as spiritual and holistic as possible under the circumstances. I would be in an institutional setting, but I vowed to deliver the baby without drugs. I planned to have fresh flowers and candles around the bed and carefully selected the music that would play in the background. I'd be calm and stoic and spend my labor in walking meditation holding my rosary that had been blessed by Mother Teresa. I'd survived Dwight's training sessions, so I knew I had a high tolerance for pain. Besides, how bad could it be?

Five days before my due date, I was lying on the couch trying to seduce Robin (again). He gently pushed on my belly and begged the baby to come out. I stood up to go to the bathroom and felt a trickle of liquid between my legs. I'd read about water breaking, but this didn't feel like the description. I called the doctor, who said yes, it was probably my water but that it would more than likely be a long night and I should stay put. He told me to call him when my contractions were five minutes apart.

It wasn't long before the contractions started, fast and furious. Right off the bat, they were three minutes apart. I called the doctor, who said, "Get to the hospital right now."

We jumped in a cab and I yelled, "Take us to Mt. Sinai Hospital—I'm having a baby!" It was like a scene out of a movie. The taxi driver drove like the dickens and got us there in record time. I was whisked to an examining room, where my doctor examined me and delivered the news that I had meconium aspirational syndrome, which meant the baby had had "an intestinal discharge" in utero. That's a nice way of saying that my baby had pooped inside of me. I would need to lie down during the remaining hours of my labor so that the affected amniotic fluid had less chance of getting inside the baby's lungs and poisoning him or her.

Instead of walking serenely around the halls of the hospital meditating on the arrival of my baby (we had opted not to find out the sex), I was lying flat on my back. A nurse kept coming in and offering me an epidural for the pain, which I kept refusing. The last time she came in, she said the anesthesiologist was going to bed, and it was now or never because I was getting very dilated. "Fine," I said. "Tell him to sleep well."

About half an hour later, I changed my mind. The pain was getting intense, so I rang for the nurse and told her I wanted the epidural. She said I was eight centimeters dilated and the anesthesiologist wasn't available. I freaked out: "Well, go wake his ass up!" I said. She did and when he arrived, he grumpily told Robin to leave the room. When he saw the scar from my recent back surgery he said, "I'm sorry. I can't give you an epidural because your surgery is too recent."

I lied. I said the surgery had taken place ten years before and the scar had always looked that way. I'm not sure if he believed me, but he went ahead and administered the epidural. It was a godsend.

My beautiful baby, Rachel Cheyenne, was born on October 5, 1995, at 9:05 a.m. I had an 8-pound, 6½-ounce girl who latched onto my breast immediately. I experienced those first pangs of total, unconditional love.

◆　◆　◆

Creating expectations and then feeling disappointed is a sad way to start motherhood or any other passage in your life. It's fine to have a plan in your head, but you need to be flexible enough to change course without regret. One of my mentors, the Zen Buddhist Roshi Joan Halifax, asks her students to do an exercise: "Write down the most horrendous death that you can imagine," she says. "Now write down the most ideal death that you can imagine. Now," she instructs, "tear up both pieces of paper. Because your death will probably be neither of these."

Disappointment occurs when there is attachment to outcomes. One of my favorite Sutras is 1.12: *abhyasa-vairagyabhyam tan-nirodhah*. My understanding of it is: Practice diligently without attachment to the fruits of your actions. This kind of effort without expectation trains the mind to stay rooted in the present moment. If we practice hip openers every day for years, we may still never be able to get our leg behind our head. Can we find tranquility in our daily practice and not be disappointed if we never attain mastery of a certain pose?

In life, expectations create a seesaw of satisfaction and disappointment. Most of us have a checklist of "I'll be happy when I have a perfect spouse, career, house, etc." Ironically, we can experience disappointment when we attain these things. It's like being a kid on Christmas morning. I thought if I only had an Easy-Bake Oven I'd be the happiest girl in the world. I got my oven and was thrilled for about twelve hours. Then I needed something else to make me happy.

I had an expectation about giving birth, and I was disappointed when it didn't turn out the way I had fantasized. We all have small daily desires. Something as insignificant as expecting ripe avocados at the market, then finding they're all hard, can make us irritable and impatient.

When you count on a future-based result, you're not living fully in the moment. Expectation can keep you locked in a narrow tunnel with no broader vision.

Joy is right here, right now. The key is mindfulness, noticing when your expectations have taken you out of the present and made you unhappy.

Another expectation I created before Rachel was born was to return to work as quickly as possible. I thought I could do it all. I had no idea what I was in for. I dieted and worked my ass off to get back to a size 4. Six weeks after giving birth (and taking advantage of the fact that I finally had boobs), I accepted a five-day swimsuit assignment in California. Before I left, I pumped what must have been one hundred bags of milk so Robin could feed Rachel while I was away.

The minute I got on the plane, I was miserable. During the shoot, I spent a lot of time "pumping and dumping" breast milk, which felt like flushing liquid gold down the toilet. If this was having it all, it felt lousy. By the time I got to the airport to fly home, I was in a state of near hysteria. So when I heard the announcement that my flight had been canceled due to weather in New York, I had a full-out meltdown. I started sobbing and shaking. People rushed up to ask what was wrong. "I need to breast-feed my baby!" I cried.

They must have thought I was crazy. I called my agency even though it was closed and screamed at the answering machine, "This is CK1!" (CK1 was my agency moniker.) "Put on my chart that CK1 does NOT travel anymore! Do you hear that? I will never do another trip!" I went on like a madwoman. I needed my baby on my breast, not some stupid swimsuit.

I made it back to New York and to my family. And I kept my vow. I only took day-long modeling jobs until Rachel started nursery school. I went from making $400,000 the year before she was born to $12,000 the year after. I had saved some money and we lived off that, but it was a stressful time. My obsessive work ethic was in conflict with my instinct to stay close to my baby. Unrealistic expectations had shoved me into a corner from which I had to work to extricate myself.

Yoga Sequence: Letting Go of Expectations

How many times did you hear your parents say "I expected more from you"? Just writing those words makes my shoulder and neck muscles tighten.

This sequence is about letting go of expectations—those you have for yourself or that others have for you. It focuses on releasing tension and pressure from the shoulders, head, and neck, which are areas where we carry stress. The sequence starts with big arm movements to loosen the shoulders. Even though these aren't all standard yoga poses, they incorporate parts of many asanas that unlock muscular binding, particularly in the upper body.

The mat is a laboratory on which we explore our reactions to life. When we practice asana, we can experience frustrations and disappointments about the capacities of our bodies. We create the mindfulness necessary to notice our expectations. Observation and detachment are the first steps toward stilling the fluctuations of the mind and letting go of desired outcomes.

As you go through each day, notice when and where tension creeps into your neck or shoulders. Yoga practice can address the residue of ruined expectations by helping alleviate the pain in our necks and shoulders and opening us to accept the situation as it is.

At the beginning of my classes, I ask students to put their hands together in prayer and dedicate their practice to someone. It can be a person you adore or someone you dislike. I never ask students to state an intention such as "I will focus on my breath for the entire practice," or "I won't rest in Child's Pose if I'm tired," or "I'll get my leg around my head today." These declarations can make you feel as if you've failed. So, simply dedicate your practice without expectation.

Vertical Arm Swings. Inhale, reach your arms up, and lift your head and chest (a). Exhale as you bend your knees and swing your arms down alongside your body (b), then straighten your legs and lift your head as you swing your arms up alongside your ears (c). Exhale as you bend your knees and drop your trunk toward your thighs (d). Continue alternating between these two movements, swinging your arms with abandon and changing the pace from slow to fast to slow. Do for 1 minute.

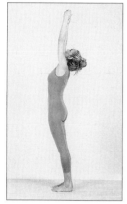
Vertical Arm Swings (a)

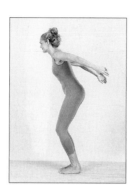
Vertical Arm Swings (b)

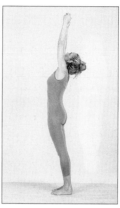
Vertical Arm Swings (c)

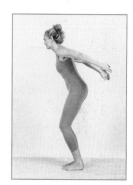
Vertical Arm Swings (d)

Helicopter Arm Swings. Take your arms out to the side and twist right and left, swinging your arms freely so your hands slap your body. Do for 1 minute.

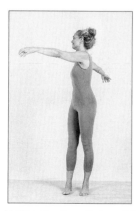
Helicopter Arm Swings (a)

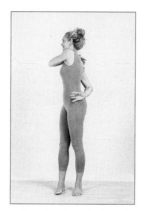
Helicopter Arm Swings (b)

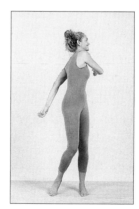
Helicopter Arm Swings (c)

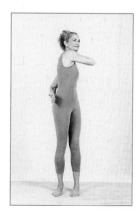
Helicopter Arm Swings (d)

Body Hug, Front and Back. Reach your arms out to the side (a), and on an exhale wrap them forward around your shoulders, left arm on top (b). Repeat 5 cycles of reaching your arms wide and hugging your body, alternating which arm is on top.

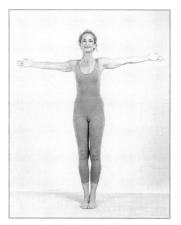

Arms Out to Side (a)

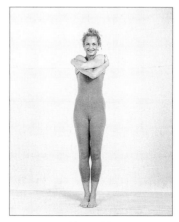

Hugs (b)

Eagle Arms (garudasana). Place your left elbow in the crook of the right, so the backs of your hands face each other. Bring your palms together if possible, or clasp your left wrist with your right hand. Drop your chin toward your chest and round your back slightly, then lift your chest and chin. Switch your arms and repeat 3 times per side.

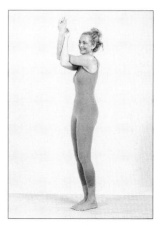

Eagle Arms

Side Bend. Inhale as you raise your arms overhead, then grab your left wrist with your right hand and side bend to the right, lifting your head and chest into a slight backbend (a). Exhale as you lean your torso laterally to the right, ears in line with upper arms (b). Then drop your chin to your chest (c). Stretch actively along your left side, and after a few breaths, move back into a side backbend (d). Stay for a few more breaths, then inhale back to upright. Switch sides, then stand in Mountain Pose.

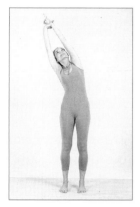
Side Bend with a
Slight Backbend (a)

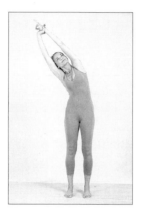
Side Bend (b)

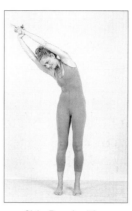
Side Bend with a
Slight Forward Bend (c)

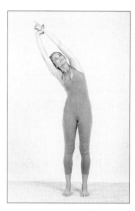
Backbend with a
Slight Side Bend (d)

Inhale and lift your arms up into **Chair Pose (utkatasana)** (a), then exhale and fold forward over straight legs into **Standing Forward Bend Variation** (b), arms reaching behind your back. Interlace your fingers and reach your arms away from your back, head dangling. Hold for 2 breaths, then inhale, bend your knees deeply, and lift your arms alongside your ears to Chair Pose. Exhale and fold forward again, changing the interlace of your fingers. Repeat 4 times (2 times for each interlace). Finish in **Mountain Pose** (c).

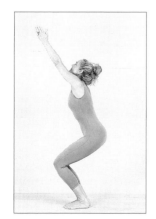
Chair Pose (a)

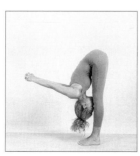
Standing Forward Bend
Variation (b)

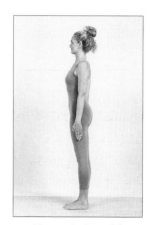
Mountain Pose (c)

Locust Variation (shalabhasana). Lie on your belly, forehead on the floor, as you reach your arms forward and perch your fingertips on a block at its lowest height. Stay for 10 breaths, then, if possible, raise the block to its middle height for another 10 breaths. Finish by moving your buttocks back onto your heels.

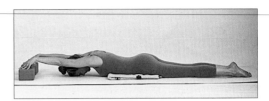

Locust Variation

Wide-Knee Child's Pose with Block (balasana). With spread knees and big toes touching each other, lengthen your torso and arms forward, pressing a block between your hands (a). Inch your elbows as far forward as you can, then bend them to swing the block overhead to touch your shoulder blades (b). Repeat 9 times, then clasp your hands behind your back and inhale to lift your hips and roll onto the crown of your head. Round your back fully into **Rabbit Pose (shashasana)** (c), change the interlace of your fingers, and repeat. Exhale, lower your buttocks back to your heels, grab your feet, and lift your hips as you roll onto the crown of your head (d). Repeat one more time. Exhale, return to Wide-Knee Child's Pose, rest your chin on the blocks (e), and walk your hands forward as far as possible.

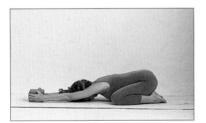

Wide-Knee Child's Pose
with Block (a)

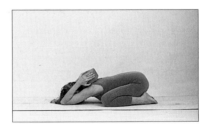

Wide-Knee Child's Pose
with Block over Shoulder (b)

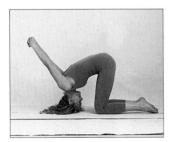

Rabbit Pose (c)

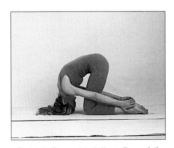

Rabbit Pose Holding Feet (d)

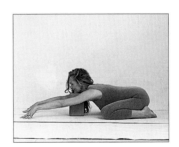

Wide-Knee Child's Pose
with Chin on Block (e)

Bent-Knee Downward-Facing Dog (adho mukha shvana-sana). Tuck your toes under and lift your hips into Downward-Facing Dog with slightly bent knees for 5 breaths. Step your right foot then left foot forward between your hands and stand in Mountain.

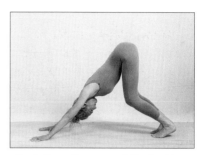

Bent-Knee Downward-Facing Dog

Pyramid Pose Preparation (parshvottanasana preparation). Press your palms behind your back or hold opposite elbows behind your back (a). Step your left foot back and plant your left heel, then lift your chest up and over your back leg and open the front of your body into **Pyramid Preparation** (b). Come back to neutral and step the right foot next to the left in Mountain Pose. Keep your palms together behind your back or place the other elbow on top and take a big step back with the right foot and plant the right heel firmly on the ground and lift your chest into a backbend. Stay for 5 breaths on both sides, then step back to Mountain Pose and release your arms.

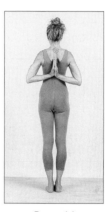

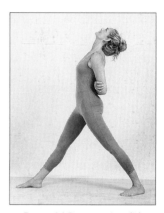

Pyramid Preparation (a)

Pyramid Preparation (b)

Eagle Pose (garudasana). Bend your knees and put your right thigh on top of your left, then tuck your right foot behind your left calf if possible. Press your left elbow in the crook of the right, so the backs of the hands face each other, then press the palms together or hold your left wrist with your right hand. Bend your knees a bit more and lift your elbows, gazing past your wrists. Stay for 5 breaths and switch sides. Then return to Mountain Pose.

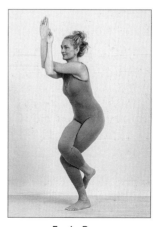

Eagle Pose

Volcano Pose (urdhva hastasana). Inhale, reach your arms up, then exhale and fold forward. Inhale, step your left foot back, then exhale and step your right foot back to Downward-Facing Dog. Come to kneel, then sandwich your left knee behind your right and part the shins to sit in between your feet.

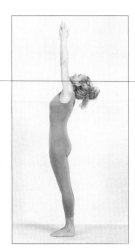

Volcano Pose

Cow Face (gomukhasana). Reach your left arm up, then bend your elbow and reach the hand as far down between the shoulder blades as possible, palm facing the torso. Internally rotate your right arm and bend it to slide your forearm and hand as high up your back as you can, palm facing out. Clasp fingers (or a strap between your hands), then lean forward any amount. Hold for 5 breaths, then reverse your arms and legs to change sides. Straighten your legs to sit in Staff Pose.

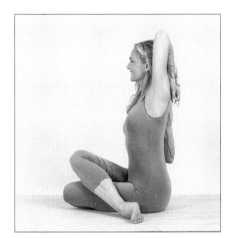

Cow Face Pose

Shoulder Stretch (purvottanasana variation). With your palms on the floor behind you, fingers toward buttocks, scoot yourself as far forward as you can, elbows bent back, chin into chest. Hold for 5 breaths, then slide back to sit up.

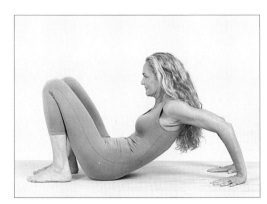

Shoulder Stretch

Reverse Tabletop (purvottanasana variation). Bend your knees and lift your torso and thighs so they are parallel to the floor, heels directly under knees, hands directly under shoulders, head neutral or dropped back. Raise and lower 3 times, holding for 2 breaths each time.

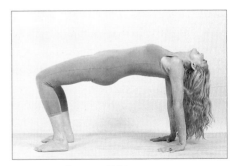

Reverse Tabletop

Easy Pose with Side Bend (sukhasana). Cross your right shin in front of your left, fingertips tented on either side of your body. Drop your right ear to your shoulder as you walk your fingertips to the right and stretch your left arm over your ear. Then turn your head to look under your left arm as you arch into a slight backbend. Stay for 5 breaths, inhale, and reverse arms and legs to repeat.

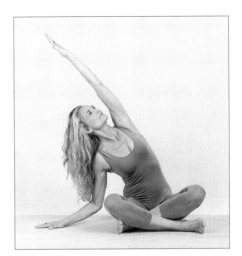

Easy Pose with Side Bend

Easy Pose with a Twist. Place your right shin in front of your left and take your left hand to your right knee and your right arm behind your back as you twist to the right. Hold for 5 breaths, then change arms and legs and twist to the left.

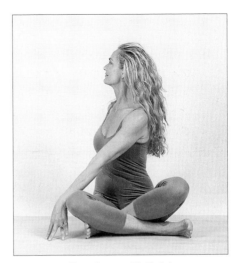

Easy Pose with Twist

Bridge Pose (setu bandha). Lie down on your back, knees bent, feet on the floor hip distance apart and as close to your buttocks as possible. Inhale, lift your hips, interlace your fingers underneath your torso, and inch your shoulders a little closer together. Press your shoulders into the floor and stay for 5 breaths. Lower with an exhalation. Change the interlace of your fingers and lift up again, holding for another 5 breaths. Lower down to the floor.

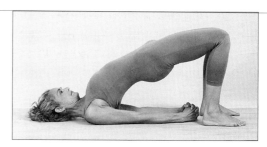

Bridge Pose

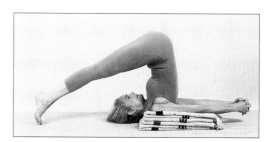

Plow Pose (a)

Plow Pose (halasana). Stack 2 or 3 folded blankets and lie with your shoulders on the blankets and your head on the mat. Your neck should not touch the blanket or the mat. Swing your legs back and over your head and rest your toes on the floor (a) or on a bolster (b) or on a chair (c), whichever makes it easy on your neck and frees the breath. Stay for 10 breaths. Slowly roll out of Plow, keeping your head back so it doesn't whiplash forward when the legs and torso touch down. Slowly slide off the blankets, lie on your back, and place your hands on your belly. Watch 5 cycles of breath.

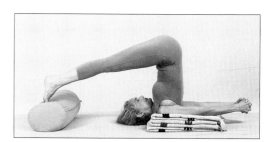

Plow Pose with Bolster (b)

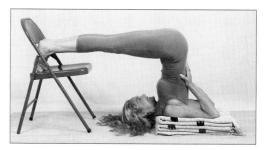

Modified Plow Pose with Chair (c)

Final Relaxation (shavasana). Place a blanket under your neck for support so that your chin is not higher than your forehead. Place a bolster under your knees and stay for 5 minutes.

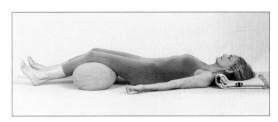

Final Relaxation

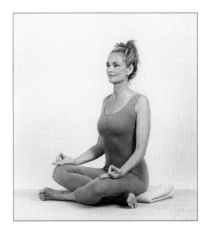

Meditation

Meditation (dhyana). Sit cross-legged with your head floating over the support of your legs and the lift of your chest. Practice watching the breath and noticing when your mind wanders. With a smile come back to observing the breath. Stay for 3 minutes.

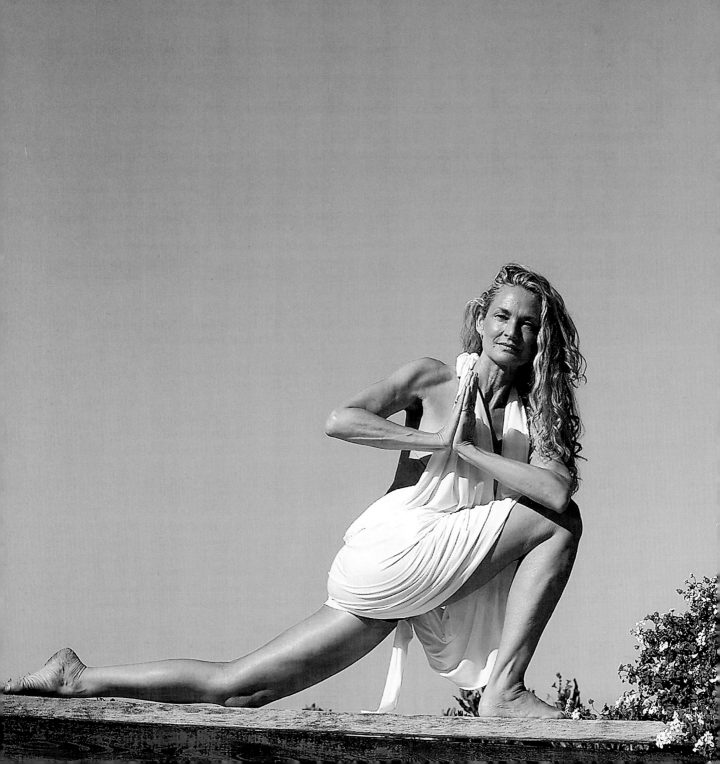

Chapter 11

TRUTH

Come out here where the roses have opened.
Let soul and world meet.

—"Empty," Rumi

After climbing up four flights of stairs that smelled like cat piss in a rundown building in the East Village of Manhattan, I reached a purple studio where I was met by the musty scent of Nag Champa incense and the sound of chanting in a language I didn't recognize. The room was bustling, colorful, and crowded with tattooed people in short shorts and tank tops—it felt like a secret club where something special was going on, and I wanted to be part of it. I put on my yoga clothes in the small changing room where an orange sari hung as a makeshift door and took my place on a mat. I'd been taking yoga classes on and off for a couple of years, but I was about to go to the next level.

This was my first visit to Jivamukti, a yoga studio I had been hearing about from friends. The founders were a couple named Sharon Gannon and David Life—both avant-garde artists who had moved to New York City, discovered yoga, traveled to India to study, and on returning opened their own studio in 1984. A *jivanmukti* is a human being who has achieved enlightenment and lives to benefit others—thus, Jivamukti Yoga. An altar at the front of the room held pictures of Sharon and David's gurus, mentors, and sources of inspiration. When I spotted a photo of Bob Dylan, I knew that I was in the right place.

The ethereal Sharon Gannon, wrapped in an Indian shawl, took her seat in the front of the room and started to chant "*Lokah samastah sukhino bhavantu*"—a Sanskrit prayer meaning "May all beings everywhere be happy and free." She added to the translation, "And may the thoughts, words, and actions of my own life contribute in some way to that happiness and to that freedom for all."

As she swayed and played a small keyboard instrument called a harmonium, she seemed to lose herself in the prayer. After she chanted a line in Sanskrit, the class would chant it back to her. This chanting is called *kirtan*, meaning "call and response." I've always considered myself tone deaf and was timid at first, but as the energy rose in the room, I found myself belting out the prayer. Amazingly, no one turned to look at the new girl, singing off-key, high on *kirtan*. When the chanting ended, the room went completely quiet. Then Sharon launched into a dharma talk (a spiritual lesson) about society's cruelty to animals and that as our fellow beings, animals deserve to be happy and free. She used their plight to teach the yoga ethic of *ahimsa*—nonviolence.

Then the class started. Sweet, beautiful Sharon—who was probably all of ninety pounds—proceeded to kick our asses. Within ten minutes, and after what seemed like a hundred sun salutations, I was slipping and sliding in my own sweat. Just when I was losing steam, the music started up. I couldn't believe it. Bob Dylan was singing "Knockin' on Heaven's Door"! This yoga thing must have been invented for me.

At one point during the class, David Life, who looked like a cross between a rock star and a *saddhu*, gave me a hands-on adjustment. He assisted me into a deep twist with his confident, experienced hands, and I trusted him. I rolled out of the building completely wrung out, but before I left I bought a tee-shirt with the Jivamukti snake logo. I was hooked.

✦ ✦ ✦

Sharon and David passed along to their students lessons they had learned from their own gurus. They were devoted to Swami Nirmalananda, a gentle man who had spent twelve years in noble silence and had a sweet message about being kind and serving the world. David and Sharon also studied with Guruji Pattabhi Jois, who codified and popularized the Ashtanga Vinyasa System.

As a couple, they were interested in social, political, and cultural change, and they put yoga into a context that made their students feel they could make a difference. Jivamukti offered asana and meditation classes, as well as the study of ancient yogic texts and Sanskrit chanting. The asana practice is rigorous and sweaty and meant to purify. Jivamukti classes are a combination of a vinyasa flow, chanting, rock and roll music, spiritual teaching, and meditation. Jivamukti Yoga holds that students have to be willing to promote the happiness of all beings if they want to realize their own full capacity for joy. David and Sharon encourage students to become vegetarian because it creates less harm to the earth and other beings.

Each class would begin with a dharma talk in which Sharon, David, or whoever was teaching the class would reflect on the topic of the month. The talks resonated with me even if they occasionally challenged my beliefs and pissed me off. I had a hard time wrapping my head around the idea that a mouse's life is as important as a child's, but the talks made me think. Sharon and David would tell us that yoga was for everyone; it wasn't a religion, but it could enhance whichever religion a person might affiliate with.

I found it rewarding to be learning so much. Modeling had always frustrated me, because it didn't offer an opportunity to grow intellectually. The older you got, the less valuable you became. In the yoga world, I didn't have to lie about my age because no one asked or cared. I could study and make progress by taking classes and reading books about the art of yoga.

I also started going to the *kirtans* that were held every Wednesday night. At these gatherings, Sharon, David, or a guest would chant in call-and-response for hours. It always became ecstatic. Sometimes I would dress in a sari and hand out what was called *prassad*, nuts or dried fruit that had been blessed by the vibration of the chanting. (Finally, I got to be the altar boy that I'd always wanted to be.)

I found comfort in yoga's commonalities with the Catholic Church: the incense, the candles, the altar, music, and the dharma talks. I've always loved the Indian aesthetic: the bright colors, the sensual shapes, even down to the details of the tassels, little bells on pillows, and anything gilded. My yoga studios today are decorated with gold-leaf ceilings, colorful walls, and ornate lights.

Yoga at Jivamukti fit my bill on every level. It provided the devotion of prayer, the endorphins of running, and the altered state of drugs, as well as a community of people who felt similar moral responsibilities in the world. Yoga pointed me in the direction of insight without the harm of drugs. As I became more involved at Jivamukti, my identity gradually shifted from model to yogi. I began digging into the quintessential yoga questions: *Who am I? Am I this body? Am I my emotions? Am I an individual, or am I a part of a greater whole?*

All my life, I'd been running away. It was time to stop. I needed to become intimate with whatever I was avoiding. When I think about this, I'm reminded of one of my favorite passages from Arthur Miller's play *After the Fall*: "I dreamed I had a child, and even in the dream I saw it was my life, and it was an idiot, and I ran away. But it always crept onto my lap again, clutched at my clothes. Until I thought, if I could kiss it, whatever in it was my own, perhaps I could sleep. And I bent to its broken face, and it was horrible . . . but I kissed it. I think one must finally take one's life in one's arms."

I was starting to settle into who I was rather than who others wanted or needed me to be—or who I needed to be to gain their approval. As a daughter, I had wanted to fix my mother's sadness by being perfect. As a model, I wanted to become the image that art directors asked me to be on the set. As a woman, I tried to be what Robin wanted. If I exercised enough, studied enough, dressed perfectly enough, made enough money, was a good enough lover and conversationalist, the other people in my life would be happy. And then, so would I.

It's not uncommon for women to put themselves on a scale (literally and metaphorically) to see if we add up. But when we take charge of ourselves and stop trying to become something that others want us to be, a significant shift takes place. Not only does internal turmoil lessen, but others can feel our honesty and genuineness shining through. It also inspires others to be authentic.

Thus, yoga also has the potential to wreak havoc on relationships. As your perspective shifts, so do your responses. In relationships, there's often an unwritten rule that we play our assigned roles. If I say this, it pushes a button in you and you will respond in a predictable way. The game changes when we become aware of our habitual responses. As Mr. Iyengar always said, "If you don't want your life to change, don't get on the mat."

◆   ◆   ◆

In 1996, I picked up the application for Jivamukti's eight-hundred-hour teacher-training program. It took me six months to fill it out; I procrastinated because I knew it would affect my life greatly and I didn't know if I was ready for that. I also knew it was a serious commitment, and not just in hours. Sharon and David expected a lot from their trainees. David said that most yoga teachers didn't live the principles that they were teaching, for example, lying to your spouse because you want to avoid conflict.

Sharon used to say to us, "How you treat others will determine how others treat you. How others treat you will determine how you see yourself. How you see yourself will determine who you are."

David and Sharon always honored the teachers who informed their study and encouraged us to broaden our own study. During the training, we were required to take a month of Pattabhi Jois yoga (rigorous ashtanga vinyasa), which meant a two-hour class six days a week for four weeks. We were also required to take a month of Iyengar yoga (slower, more alignment-based) classes.

Teacher training required that we live and breathe yoga. The history and depth of yoga was being introduced to me through the seminal texts: the sutras, the *Bhagavad Gita*, the *Upanishads*, and the *Hatha Yoga Pradipika*. We also studied basic Sanskrit. Each of us kept a notebook of our writings. All of this study was elementary given the vastness of yoga's lineage, philosophy, and physical practice, but I gave it my all.

We learned about the *kriyas*, which are yoga cleansing practices that range from sharp breath exhalations (*kapalabhati*) to scrubbing your skin with a rough brush to cleaning out your nasal passages with a neti pot, to more extreme practices such as inserting gauze down your throat, as well as other techniques to cleanse the intestines. I had a seizure on the day we were doing some of the *kriyas* and couldn't participate in the cleansings—but have practiced many of them over the years. They can be a part of the process of uncovering the true self, hidden beneath the impurities.

One day during the middle of the course, I went to Sharon and David's office, which was at the beautiful new Jivamukti studio on Lafayette Street in NoHo. They invited me in as if they'd been expecting me, and looked at each other as if they knew what I had come to say. I nervously informed them that I was not going to become a yoga teacher but that I would continue taking the training to deepen my practice. Then I launched into my laundry list of why I would never become a teacher.

"First," I said, "I'm shy, and talking in front of a group of people is not my thing. Second, I'm tone deaf and won't be able to lead chants. Third, I'm slightly dyslexic and I can't mirror a class." (When you're facing a roomful of students and demonstrating a pose you describe the opposite of what you are doing, as if the student were looking into a mirror.) "Fourth, I have epilepsy and if I had a seizure while teaching, it would traumatize the students and embarrass me."

They listened patiently while I talked. Then they nodded and said, "Well, those are the reasons you *should* be a teacher. If you're going to stand in front of a class, tone deaf, and chant, that's going to be inspiring to people." They told me that as we face our own fears, we give others the courage to face theirs, too. They went down my list and explained why these were all reasons to teach. Despite their arguments, at the end of the meeting they looked as if they had accepted my not-so-graceful bowing out, and I left feeling relieved.

At three o'clock that afternoon, my phone rang. It was Sharon. "Colleen, you're teaching my six-fifteen class tonight," she said. "It's sold out, and I'll be taking the class."

I panicked. The 6:15 class was the busiest of the day and the one that the most high-powered New Yorkers attended. They would be expecting Sharon, of course, and they would be getting . . . me. Ugh. To this day, I still remember the sequence I taught. David and Sharon threw me into the deep end of the pool, because they knew that blindsiding me was the only way I would ever get in front of a class.

Teaching that evening produced a whole new kind of high. Afterward, my body was buzzing from adrenaline and relief. I went from being furious at Sharon and David to being sublimely grateful. They were right. I had faced my fears and succeeded in teaching a decent class.

As part of the training, Sharon and David would often invite outside teachers to give workshops. That year, 1998, Rodney Yee was one of the guest teachers, and his class was mandatory. I rushed to get there from a modeling job and arrived a little late. There was one mat free at the front of the room. His instruction was meticulous and poetic—and the students were lapping it up. Still, something about him made me feel I couldn't be in the same room with him. It was a visceral reaction. For the first time in my life, I got up and left a yoga class. I went to David and Sharon. "I'm so sorry," I said, "but I can't stay in the same room with that man. If you want to fail me for not attending you can." They didn't fail me, and it would be several years until I understood what my reaction was all about.

At the end of the training, our class of twenty-odd students graduated as Jivamukti-certified yoga teachers. The ceremony was beautiful. I still keep the photograph of David and Sharon handing me my diploma on my altar in my home studio. It was a cherished moment. I had never worked as hard or felt that I had accomplished something so significant.

Sharon and David offered me a regular 8:00 a.m. class on Wednesdays. I was honored and accepted. With Rachel in nursery school, I had begun modeling again. My career was picking up steam, and my agency worked around my yoga commitments as much as it could. The first day I taught, there were eight students in class. I had stayed up all night rehearsing every word and was exhausted. Halfway through the class I walked smack into a column in the middle of the room and gashed my forehead. Bleeding, I grabbed some tissues and applied pressure to the wound. I stayed fairly calm and put the students in Child's Pose, Downward-Facing Dog, and any other pose I could think of in which they couldn't look up and see me. After class, I rushed to the doctor and got stitches.

In those days, I was trying to balance being a mother, yoga teacher, model, and wife—in that order. For the first time I felt I was finding my voice in the world. As a result, I threw all my energy into the parts of my life where I was being validated.

I loved teaching and started thinking about opening a yoga studio outside the city. Robin and I had spent time on Shelter Island, but it seemed like the Hamptons would make more sense businesswise. I knew of a Jivamukti teacher, Jessica Bellofatto, who had graduated the year before me and was giving classes in the Hamptons. I liked her and her teaching style. "What do you think about opening a yoga studio together?" I asked.

"Sure!" she said.

Each of us took $1,500 out of the ATM. We'd decided on the name Yoga Shanti—*shanti* means "peace," "tranquility," "bliss." An artist designed the logo and we rented space, a small apartment next to Murf's Backstreet Tavern in Sag Harbor, a quaint, unpretentious town between the Hamptons and Shelter Island. The studio could hold twenty-two mats with about two inches of space between them. On October 4, 1999, the day before Rachel's fourth birthday, we excitedly hung the Yoga Shanti shingle.

Although a few individuals were teaching classes in the Hamptons, there was no formal yoga studio in the area, and word spread fast. We outgrew our space in eighteen months and moved to a spot behind a kite shop on Main Street. We were excited that the room held thirty-five mats—thirteen more than our first space! We stayed there for several years, and then moved to a bigger street-front store with room for forty-five mats. Eventually, Jessica and I parted ways, but I continued with the Yoga Shanti studio that exists today—a beautiful, shimmering jewel box that sits on a hill one block behind Sag Harbor's main drag. We squeeze seventy-five mats into this yoga beehive, which is home to the many yogis we are blessed to teach.

A yoga class is always fascinating. All kinds of people show up for all different reasons. There's the man whose wife just walked out on him without explanation. There's the addict struggling to stay clean. There's the woman who wants a nice butt. There are those who use yoga as an anti-aging tool. There's the person with low self-esteem who can't understand why he or she is still in an abusive relationship. There's the high-powered businesswoman looking for stress relief. There are people who are lonely, hurt, or seeking community. There are also those who are simply curious.

Yoga practice addresses the question *Who am I?* But it doesn't deliver the answer on a silver platter. Getting there is a journey that always takes effort, honesty, and plenty of soul searching. When you uncover something you've spent decades burying, it can be pretty smelly. I am still peeling back layers of shame, guilt, repression, sadness, and anger, yet I am willing to show up on my mat every day. Just when I think I've peeled back a layer and am getting somewhere, another one appears—and another. The answer lies within, and yoga moves me in the right direction.

David Life always said that, as teachers, we had a responsibility to our students to walk our talk. The possibility of helping or inspiring people to find their own way was a privilege. I needed to step up to the plate and do the work.

Besides running a yoga studio in Sag Harbor, I was teaching two classes a week at Jivamukti in New York City. (Sharon and David had given me my own 6:15 p.m. class.) Between modeling and teaching, I spent a lot of time on the bus from the Hamptons to Manhattan. Yoga Shanti didn't bring in enough money for us to live on, and I wasn't ready to give up modeling. In fact, I had moved into a new category of "middle-aged" modeling, which was relatively new ground for the industry. Just before my fortieth birthday, I was giving a dharma a talk about truthfulness. I talked about taking off masks rather than putting them on. It was time to listen to my own teaching. So on my fortieth birthday, I called my closest model friends and told them I had a confession: my true age was forty, not thirty-seven; I was finally coming out of the closet. Initially, my friends were confused and upset. I regretted my honesty at first, but soon I felt liberation and relief. As yoga says, adherence to *satya*, or truthfulness, will set you free.

Yoga Sequence: Practicing Truthfulness

At Jivamukti, we investigated the practice of *satya*, the yoga precept (or *yama*) of truthfulness. We start with small steps, becoming conscious of the little lies we tell almost without knowing. A small secret or lie can have great power. Lying about my age for so long was like carrying a weight on my chest. A lie is never isolated; you need more lies to cover up the initial one. The energy required to hold up the mask of untruth is exhausting and it alienates us from ourselves.

Yoga breaks through our lies and defenses with the intense heat of practice. Asanas create an internal combustion that affects us physically, psychologically, and emotionally. This purification is called *tapas*, which is translated as "heat," "glow," "discipline," or "austerity." *Tapas* burns impurities that impede us and keep us separate from the divine. Shedding the layers of false self requires dedication to your practice. The dedication isn't only the effort you bring to a particular pose—it's also the consistency of getting on your mat, of telling one less lie, of letting go of one more bit of anger or resentment every day. Dharma talks and yoga scriptures introduce a different kind of fire, one that tests your beliefs. Philosophical friction creates heat. Yoga says the liberated self is buried within us. I love the analogy of the musk deer that roots around for a beautiful smell that is bedeviling it—never realizing that the smell is its own.

This is a heat-building vinyasa practice that is intended to burn impurities. I've built on the template of the first Jivamukti class I taught seventeen years ago. I began with the mantra of the classic Buddhist teaching, *Prajna paramita*, the Heart Sutra: *Gate gate para gate para sam gate bodhi swaha*. The translation is, "Gone, gone, way gone, beyond gone, awake, so be it." I talked about how in yoga we work to get beyond our stories, our constructed identities, our likes and dislikes, until we arrive at the pure state of yoga, which is truth.

Shining Skull Breath (kapalabhati) with Reverse Tabletop variation. Sit in Easy Pose (sukhasana), take 3 normal breaths, and then inhale to a comfortable level and begin sharp, rapid exhalations by pumping the belly. Keep your exhales active, your inhales passive, and the breath audible in the nostrils, not the throat. After 16 pumpings, drop your chin toward your chest and take 3 smooth breaths with a relaxed belly (a). Inhale, lift your head, and begin another cycle of kapalabhati. Then lean back on your hands and lift your hips halfway to **Reverse Tabletop** (b). Change the cross of your shins and lower into Easy Pose for 2 more rounds. This exercise heats the body and cleans the cobwebs out of your head. Now move onto your hands and knees.

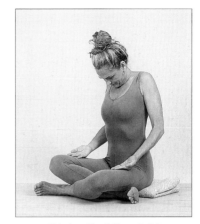

Shining Skull Breath (a)

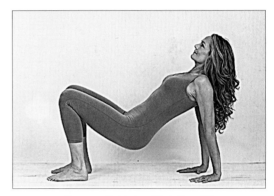

Reverse Tabletop Variation (b)

As you inhale, tilt your pelvis into a backbend, lifting your head to look forward and up into **Cow Pose** (a); then exhale and hunch your back, pressing your tailbone toward the floor and dipping your head to look at your belly in **Cat Pose** (b). Repeat 5 times. Cat-Cow is a perfect preparation for Sun Salutations, since they are composed of alternating back- and forward bends. From Cow Pose, lift your hips to **Bent-Knee Downward-Facing Dog** (c). Pedal your legs 4 times, then walk your feet between your hands. Bend and straighten your legs 4 times. Look forward, put your hands on your hips, and come to stand in Mountain Pose.

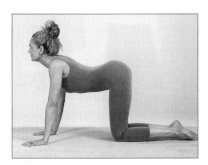

Cow Pose (a)

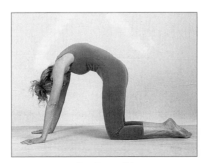

Cat Pose (b)

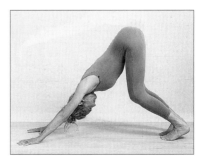

Bent-Knee Downward-Facing Dog (c)

Sun Salutation variation (surya namaskar). Inhale, lift your arms up over your head (a), and on your exhale, fold forward (b). Inhale, bend your knees, and look forward (c), then exhale and step your right foot back to a lunge (d). Inhale, lift your chest, exhale, and step your left foot back to **Downward-Facing Dog** (e). Set your knees on the floor, inhale into Cow (f), and exhale as you pull your hips back to **Downward-Facing Dog** (g). Stay 2 breaths, then walk your feet forward. Inhale, look forward, exhale, and fold into a deep **Standing Forward Bend** (h). Salute the sun again (i), this time stepping your left, then your right foot into **Downward-Facing Dog** (j). Then inhale to Plank (k) and exhale as you lower yourself to the floor. Inhale to pull your chest forward and up to a low **Cobra** (l). Exhale and pull back to **Downward-Facing Dog** (m); stay for 2 breaths. Walk your feet forward, inhale, and look up (n), then exhale, and fold forward (o). Take a few breaths, then lift to **Mountain Pose** (p).

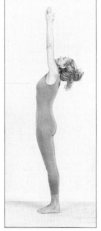

Arms Overhead (a)

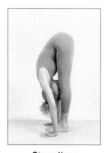

Standing
Forward Bend (b)

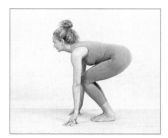

Extended Standing
Forward Bend (c)

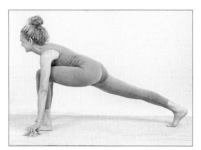

Lunge (d)

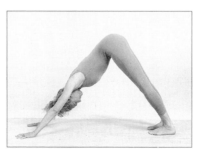

Downward-Facing Dog (e)

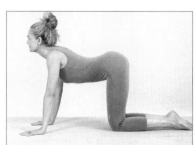

Cow Pose (f)

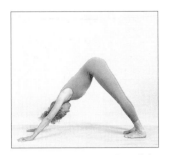

Downward-Facing Dog (g)

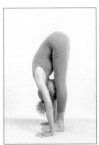

Standing
Forward Bend (h)

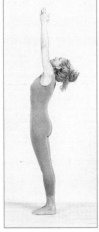

Arms Overhead (i)

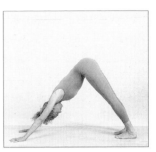

Downward-Facing Dog (j)

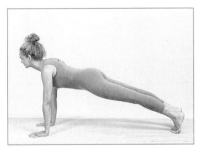

Plank (k)

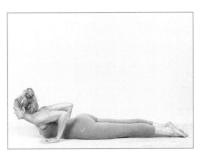

Cobra Prep (l)

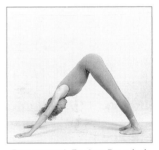

Downward-Facing Dog (m)

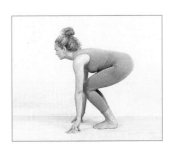

Extended Standing
Forward Bend (n)

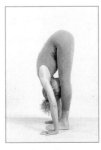

Standing
Forward Bend (o)

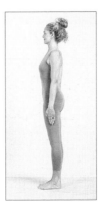

Mountain Pose (p)

Vinyasa Flow with Standing Poses. From **Mountain Pose** (a) inhale and reach your arms up toward the ceiling (b). Exhale and fold forward into **Standing Forward Bend** (c). Inhale, bend your knees, and look forward (d); exhale and step your left foot back into **Lunge** (e). Plant your left heel and spiral up to **Warrior II** (f), then reach your left hand down your left leg to **Reverse Warrior** (g). Bring your hands to the floor, then step back to **Downward-Facing Dog** (h). Take your right knee to the floor, shift onto your inner left foot and right arm, and raise your left arm up to **Side Plank Variation** (i). Stay for 3 breaths and move back to **Downward-Facing Dog** (j). Repeat the Side Plank Variation with your left knee on the floor and your right arm raised. Again, stay for 3 breaths. Then take 3 small, easy jumps forward toward your hands and walk the rest of the way to the front of your mat. Repeat steps (a) to (j), stepping your right foot back and doing Warrior II and Reverse Warrior on the other side, ending in **Downward-Facing Dog**. Inhale to Plank (k), and this time exhale to the full Side Plank (l): shift onto the outside edge of your right foot, stack the left leg on top of the right, and support yourself on the right arm (if this is difficult, repeat the bent-knee variation). Hold for 3 breaths, swing back to **Downward-Facing Dog** (m), and do Side Plank for 3 breaths on the left side. After 2 breaths in Downward-Facing Dog, inhale as you lift your right leg into the air and exhale to swing the foot forward between your hands. Ground your back heel, press your right elbow on your right thigh (or slide the hand to the floor on the outside of the right foot), opening the front torso to the left, and take your left arm up over the ear to **Extended Side Angle** (n). Stay for 3 breaths, step back to **Downward-Facing Dog** (o), then take your knees, chest, and chin to the floor (p). Lift up to **Cobra** (q) and exhale back to **Downward-Facing Dog** (r). Repeat the entire sequence on your left side. After finishing in Downward-Facing Dog, bend your knees, exhale, and lightly jump forward. Inhale, look up (s), exhale, fold forward (t). Inhale, lift your torso, and reach your arms up, then exhale into **Mountain Pose** (u).

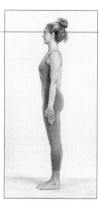

Mountain Pose (a)

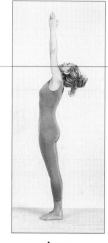

Arms Overhead (b)

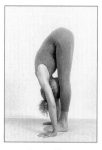

Standing Forward Bend (c)

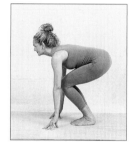

Extended Standing Forward Bend (d)

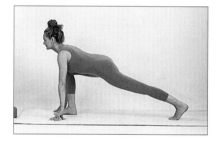

Lunge (e)

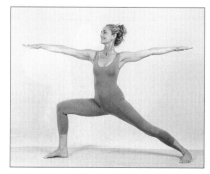

Warrior II (f)

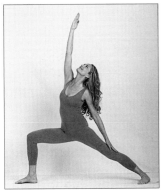

Reverse Warrior (g)

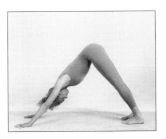

Downward-Facing Dog (h)

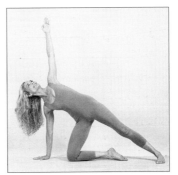

Side Plank Variation (i)

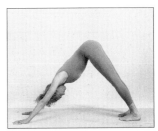

Downward-Facing Dog (j)

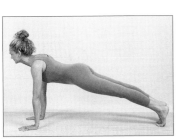

Plank (k)

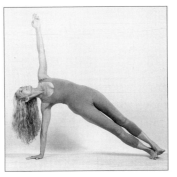

Side Plank (l)

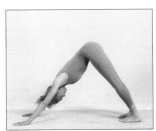

Downward-Facing Dog (m)

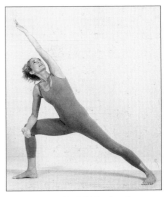

Extended Side Angle
Variation (n)

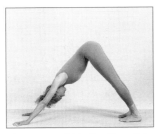

Downward-Facing Dog (o)

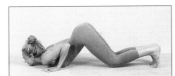

Cobra Preparation (p)

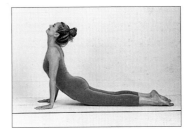

Cobra (q)

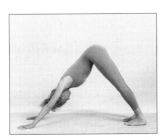

Downward-Facing Dog (r)

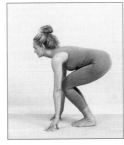

Extended Standing
Forward Bend (s)

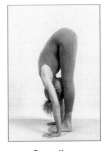

Standing
Forward Bend (t)

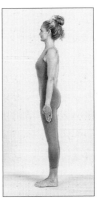

Mountain Pose (u)

Vinyasa Flow with Backbends. Inhale, bend your knees, and reach your arms up for **Chair Pose** (a). Exhale and fold forward into **Standing Forward Bend** (b). Inhale, bend your knees, and look forward (c); exhale and step your right foot back into **Lunge** (d); put your right knee down on the floor and reach your arms up, press your palms together, and drop your head back into **Crescent Lunge** (e). Stay for 3 breaths. Then take your hands to the floor, straighten your left leg, and step your right leg forward to come back to **Standing Forward Bend** (f). Step your left foot back, lower your knee, and lift to Crescent Lunge, then pull your hips back to **Downward-Facing Dog** (g). Inhale to **Plank** (h), and as you exhale, lower down to **Four-Limbed Staff Pose** (i), then inhale to **Upward-Facing Dog** (j), keeping your knees off the floor and your legs strong. Stay for 2 breaths. Exhale into **Downward-Facing Dog** (k) for 5 breaths. Step your feet forward, and lift to **Mountain Pose** (l) with an inhale.

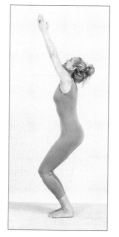

Chair Pose (a)

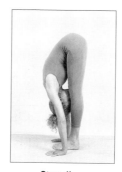

Standing
Forward Bend (b)

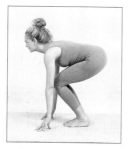

Extended Standing
Forward Bend (c)

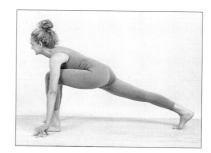

Lunge (d)

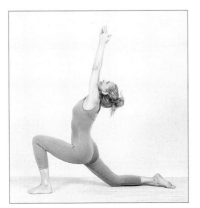

Crescent Lunge (e)

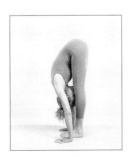

Standing
Forward Bend (f)

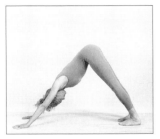

Downward-Facing Dog (g)

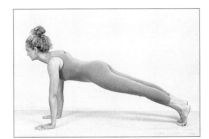

Plank (h)

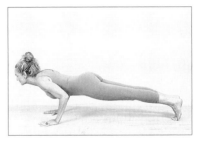

Four-Limbed Staff Pose (i)

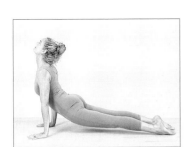

Upward-Facing Dog (j)

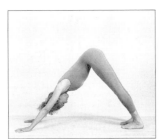

Downward-Facing Dog (k)

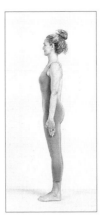

Mountain Pose (l)

Sun Salutation B (surya namaskar B). Inhale, bend your knees toward a right angle, and reach your arms up to **Chair Pose** (a). Exhale, fold forward to **Standing Forward Bend** (b). Inhale, look forward, and with an exhale, jump back to **Four-Limbed Staff Pose** (c). Inhale, sweep to **Upward-Facing Dog** (d), exhale, and move back to **Downward-Facing Dog** (e). Step your right foot forward between your hands, plant your back heel, and reach your arms up to **Warrior I** (f). Exhale, lower back down to **Four-Limbed Staff Pose** (g), inhale to **Upward-Facing Dog** (h), and exhale to **Downward-Facing Dog** (i). Step your left foot forward to **Warrior I** (j) and repeat **Four-Limbed Staff Pose** (k) to **Upward-Facing Dog** (l) and **Downward-Facing Dog** (m) and stay for 5 breaths. Jump your feet forward, bend your knees to **Chair Pose** (n), then straighten your knees as you come to stand in **Mountain Pose** (o). Repeat this cycle, but instead of jumping forward after Downward-Facing Dog, lower yourself to lie prone on the floor. Reach your arms forward and press the pads of your fingers into the floor (p). Then lift your head and upper torso into a **Locust Pose Variation** (q) for 5 breaths. Lower down with an exhale and rest, shifting your hips from side to side. Lift back to **Locust**, but this time raise your arms and legs off the floor (r). Hold for 3 breaths, lower down to rest, and repeat, lifting both the arms and legs for 3 breaths.

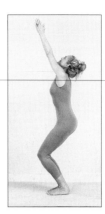

Chair Pose (a)

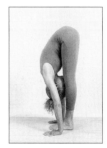

Standing Forward Bend (b)

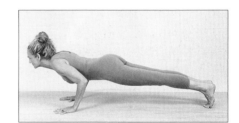

Four-Limbed Staff Pose (c)

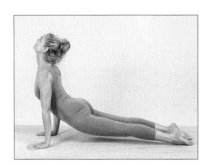

Upward-Facing Dog (d)

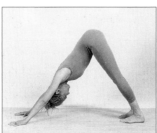

Downward-Facing Dog (e)

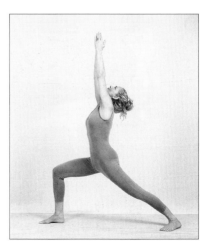

Warrior I (f)

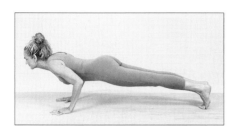
Four-Limbed Staff Pose (g)

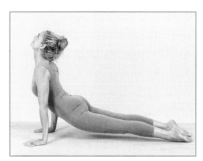
Upward-Facing Dog (h)

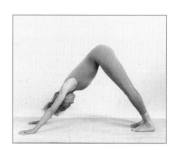
Downward-Facing Dog (i)

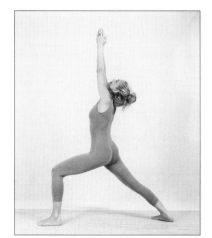
Warrior I (j)

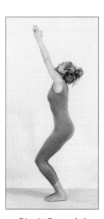
Four-Limbed Staff Pose (k)

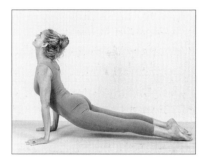
Upward-Facing Dog (l)

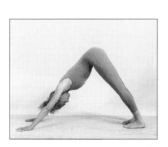
Downward-Facing Dog (m)

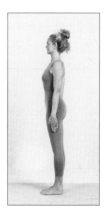
Chair Pose (n)

Mountain Pose (o)

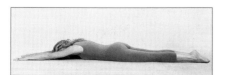
Locust Pose Preparation (p)

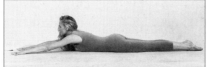
Locust Pose Variation (q)

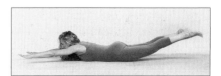
Locust Pose (r)

Hero Pose (virasana). Kneel, separate your feet slightly wider than your hips, then sit between your feet in **Hero Pose** (use a block to support the buttocks if needed) (a). Interlace your fingers and reach your arms overhead with your palms facing the ceiling (b). Change the interlace and repeat, holding for 5 breaths on each interlace. Lean back on your hands to stretch the front of your thighs in **Reclined Hero Pose Preparation** (c). Lower to your forearms on the floor behind you (d), or, if you can, lie back completely into **Reclined Hero Pose** (e). Hold for 5 breaths, then sit up and lie facedown on your mat.

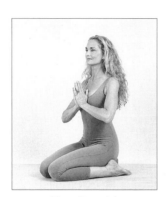

Hero Pose (a)

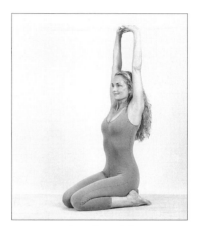

Hero Pose (b)

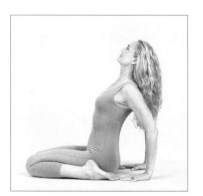

Reclined Hero Pose Preparation (c)

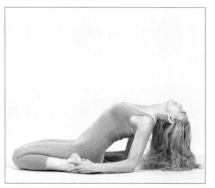

Reclined Hero Pose Variation (d)

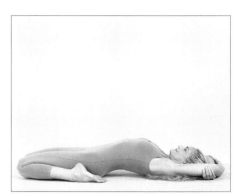

Reclined Hero Pose (e)

Bow Pose (dhanurasana). Bend your knees, bring your heels to your buttocks, and reach back to grab your ankles (a). Pulling your heels away from your buttocks, lift your thighs off the floor and sweep your chest forward and up into **Bow Pose** (b). Hold for 3 breaths, lower down, and repeat. Then come to your hands and knees and move back into **Downward-Facing Dog** for a few breaths (c). Take your knees to the floor, then swing your legs around to lie on your back.

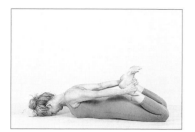

Bow Pose Preparation (a)

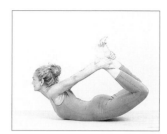

Bow Pose (b)

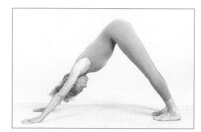

Downward-Facing Dog (c)

Upward Bow Pose (urdhva dhanurasana). Bend your knees and step your feet on the floor as close to the sit bones as possible. Press your palms on the floor alongside your ears, elbows bent, fingers pointing toward your shoulders (a). Lift your hips, push up with your legs and arms, and hold **Upward Bow** for 5 breaths (b), then lower down (c). (If this is too difficult, lift your hips and roll to the crown of your head without putting too much weight on it for 5 breaths.)

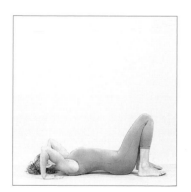

Upward Bow Preparation (a)

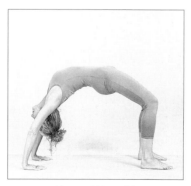

Upward Bow (b)

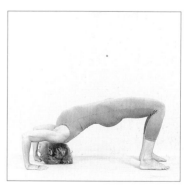

Upward Bow Variation (c)

Reclining Big Toe Pose (supta padangushthasana). Lie on your back, place a strap around the ball of your right foot, and straighten your leg toward the ceiling. Reach your left leg strongly along the floor. Hold for 8 breaths, change legs, roll to your right side, and sit up. This pose helps to bring your spine back to neutral after backbends and begins to cool you down after the heat of the vinyasa. Roll over and come to sit.

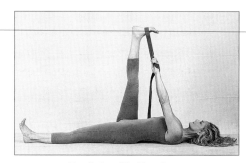

Reclining Big Toe Pose

Bound Angle Pose (baddha konasana). Sit with the soles of your feet touching, knees open to the sides. Draw your feet as close to your hips as possible. Press your hands on the floor behind your pelvis and lift your chest. Hold for 5 breaths.

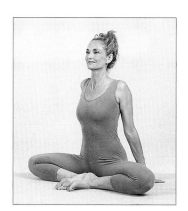

Bound Angle Pose

Wide-Legged Seated Pose (upavishtha konasana). From Bound Angle, spread your legs as wide as you can, press your hands to the floor behind you, and lift your chest. Slightly pump your legs by bending and straightening your knees 5 times, then cross your shins and pull forward to sit on your feet. The last three poses have all been neutral poses.

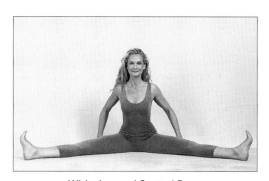

Wide-Legged Seated Pose

Child's Pose (balasana). Separate your knees and walk your hands forward to lay your torso on your thighs. After 5 breaths, slide your knees together and lift up to sit on your feet.

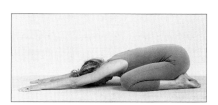

Child's Pose

Headstand or Headstand Preparation (shirshasana). *Note: Headstand is for intermediate or advanced students.* Interlace your fingers and set your forearms on a folded mat, elbows in line with shoulders. Then place the top of your head on the floor between your hands, lift your knees, and push off the ground with both feet to bring your heels to your buttocks (a); extend your legs toward the ceiling and squeeze them together (b). It's fine to use the wall for this pose, but make sure your knuckles touch the wall, and that you use your arms and your legs to lift the weight off your neck. Stay for 15 breaths. (If you are not practicing Headstand, set your arms as instructed and pull your legs back toward Downward-Facing Dog, head dangling, for 10 breaths) (c). Come down slowly and be careful not to put any strain on your neck as you bring both knees to your chest and then feet to the floor, resting in **Child's Pose** for 5 breaths (d). Cross your shins and sit down behind your feet.

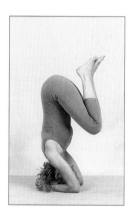

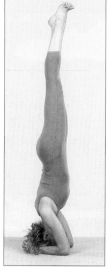

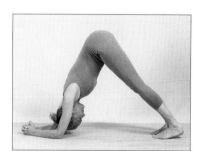

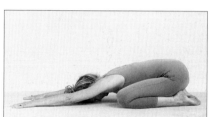

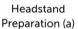
Headstand
Preparation (a)

Headstand (b)

Headstand Variation (c)

Child's Pose (d)

Reverse Tabletop (purvottanasana). Take your hands behind you and on an inhale press into your hands and feet to lift your torso as high as you can. Lower down with an exhale, then lift and lower twice more. This pose balances your shoulders after the Sun Salutations. Lie down on your back.

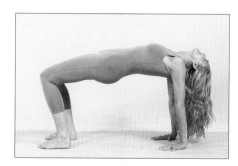
Reverse Tabletop

Supported Bridge Pose with Raised Legs (setu bandha variation). Bend your knees and lift your hips, positioning a block under your sacrum. Exhale, bend your knees into your belly, and, making sure the block is steady, reach your legs into the air (a). If your hamstrings are tight, keep your knees slightly bent. (b). Stay for 20 breaths to cool the nervous system from the heat of Headstand. Step on your feet, lift your hips, and remove the block. Lower down, and slide your legs long on the floor.

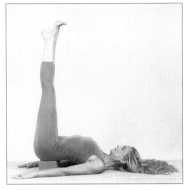
Supported Bridge Pose Variation (a)

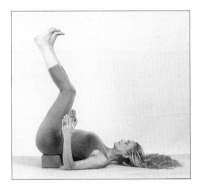
Modified Supported Bridge Pose (b)

Reclining Spinal Twist (supta matsyendrasana). Hug your right knee into your chest, stretch your left leg long, and use your left hand to draw your right knee across your torso. Hold for a few breaths, then gently rock the body from side to side. Change sides, and come to sit in Staff Pose.

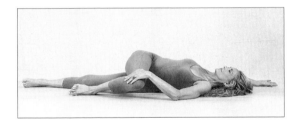
Reclining Spinal Twist

Half-Seated Spinal Twist (ardha matsyendrasana). Bend your knees to bring your feet to the floor. Slide your left foot under your right leg, bringing your left heel outside your right hip. Now step your right foot on the floor to the outside of your left thigh and twist your torso to the right. Wrap your left arm around your right knee and hug your right thigh to your chest. Hold for 5 breaths, then reverse to twist left.

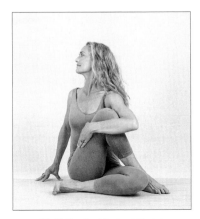
Half-Seated Spinal Twist

Star Pose (tarasana). Bring your soles together, knees out to the sides so your legs form a diamond shape. With an exhale, lean forward and rest your forehead either on a block, which is placed on your feet (a), or on your stacked, fisted hands (b). Stay for 10 breaths, then sit up in Staff Pose.

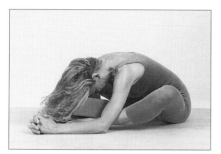

Star Pose (a)

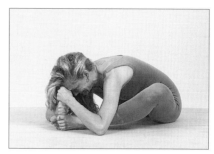

Star Pose (b)

Seated Forward Bend (pashchimottanasana). Straighten your legs and fold forward to a position that allows you to have even sensation throughout the spine. Stay for 10 breaths. Then return to Staff Pose as you inhale. Forward bending turns the mind inward, away from external stimulation as a preparation for Final Relaxation.

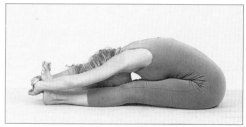

Seated Forward Bend

Plow Pose (halasana). From Staff Pose, exhale and roll onto your back. Lie down with your shoulders on a stack of firmly folded blankets and your head on the mat. Your neck should not touch the blanket or mat. Swing your legs up and over your head, taking your toes to the floor (a) or to a bolster behind you (b). Stay for 10 breaths. (If this pose is difficult, lie on your back and hug your knees into your belly, then lower your legs back down slowly.) Come to lie on your back.

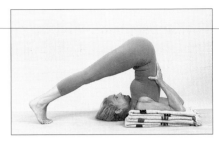

Plow Pose (a)

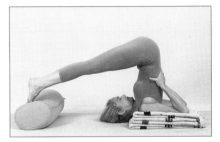

Modified Plow Pose with Bolster(b)

Happy Baby Pose. Bend your knees and hold the outer edges of your feet. Press the thighs toward the floor and keep the soles of your feet parallel to the ceiling. Hold for 8 breaths, then lower your feet to the mat.

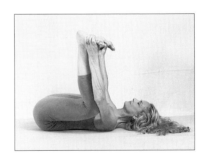

Happy Baby Pose

Constructive Rest. Widen your feet to the outside edges of your mat, drop your knees together, and place your hands on your belly; watch the rise and fall of your breath. Let the rhythm lull you into relaxation. Stay for 2 minutes.

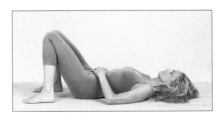

Constructive Rest

Final Relaxation (shavasana). Straighten your legs along the floor and cover yourself with a blanket to retain your body heat. Stay for 5 minutes.

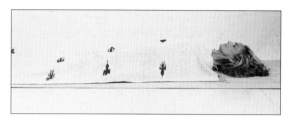

Final Relaxation

Meditation (dhyana). Sit in a comfortable cross-legged position and observe the clarity of your body and mind, as if you had just cleaned your house. Feel the expansive quality of the body that comes from ridding impurities through heat. Stay for 5 minutes.

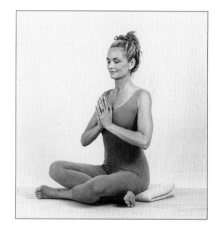

Meditation

Put your hands in prayer position and reflect on what truth you may be covering up and where lies may be stuck in your body. Breathe in and out as you say *om* three times from that place.

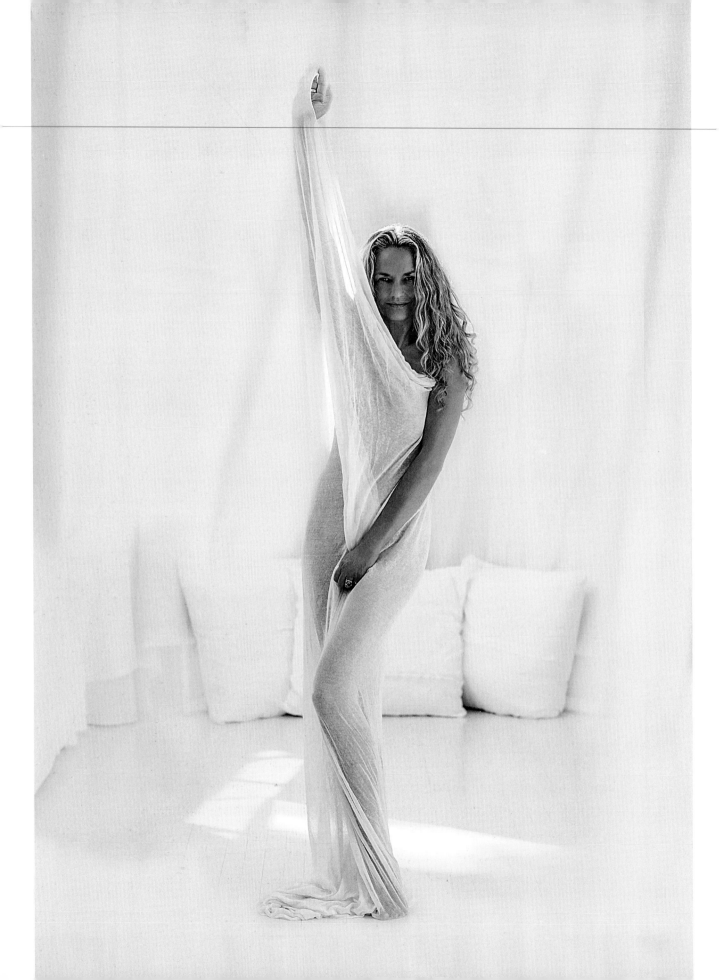

Chapter 12

LOVE

Even
After
All this time
The sun never says to the earth,
"you owe
Me."

Look
What happens
With a love like that,
It lights the
Whole
Sky.

—"The Sun Never Says," Hafiz (tr. Ladinsky)

By 2001, Robin and I had been together for almost two decades and married for twelve years. Rachel was six years old and entering the first grade. I had found my stride and rhythm in teaching, modeling, and mothering. I felt validated in every part of my life except my marriage, where I still felt stifled and stupid. The unhealthy dynamics of my relationship with Robin were so ingrained I wasn't able to see them. In my eyes, Robin was the smart one and I was the mute wage earner.

Yoga Shanti had become a hip yoga studio where we taught challenging classes to rock and roll music. We often got mentions in the New York newspapers, mainly because of the various celebrities who attended classes. I wanted to be a great teacher and build my business, and under that pressure, I began replaying my ad-olescent perfectionism. I was obsessed with planning my classes and would sit for hours with a dozen yoga books around me, writing out sequences and dharma talks, putting together the perfect playlists, and finding the ideal readings that would end my classes on the perfect note.

One day a fellow Jivamukti teacher named Rhana Harris, whom I adored, asked if I planned to attend the annual Yoga Journal Conference. When I said yes, she said, "I'm really excited about taking the full-day intensive with Rodney Yee."

"Good luck with that," I said sarcastically. "I can't stand the guy. There's barely enough space in the room for him and his ego."

In fact, I was planning to attend the conference and instead, I chose a daylong workshop with T. K. V. Desikachar, the son of Tirumulai Krishnamacharya. Krish-namacharya had been guru to some of the most influential yoga teachers of our time: B. K. S. Iyengar, Pattabhi Jois, Indra Devi, and Desikachar. To have direct contact with one of Krishnamacharya's students was an incredible opportunity. Rhana and I wanted to spend the day together at the conference, so we flipped a coin to see if I would go to Rodney's workshop with her or she would come to Desikachar's work-shop with me. I lost the coin flip and grudgingly agreed to go to Rodney's class, as long as we stayed in the back of the room and I could leave at lunchtime if I hated it.

By midday, I had to admit that Rodney was an excellent teacher. He made things I had found boring about yoga interesting and relevant. I felt clear and calm at the end of class, which I think was due to the alignment principles and specific se-quencing he taught. For the first time I really understood the Iyengar camp's edict against moving students directly from backbends to forward bends. Rodney made clear that the transition is too jarring on the nervous system, likening it to taking a glass out of the oven and putting it straight into the freezer. He also emphasized how hard it is on the intervertebral disks, which get pushed forward in backbends and backward in forward bends, and explained how to neutralize the spine instead. I left thinking I could learn a lot from this Rodney Yee. I respected him as a teacher but could still feel myself resisting him as a person.

I went home and put some of the things I'd learned into my Yoga Shanti teach-ing and practice. I had taken fastidious notes during the workshop and pored over them for hours, incorporating the concepts Rodney had taught—such as not com-promising the hip joint by linking a long series of standing poses on one side. He called this "loading the hip," and said that, for the sake of our students' hip joints, we had to stop. That is, many vinyasa teachers will teach Triangle Pose, then Extended Side Angle Pose, then Half Moon Pose, and then Standing Split—all on the right side, which gives you a good workout, but jams the hip and wears away the cartilage. I had to admit it made sense.

About a year later, one of my favorite instructors at Yoga Shanti, Heidi Michel Fokine, told me that she'd made plans to attend a weeklong training with Rodney in Albuquerque and asked me to go with her. I was intrigued enough with Rodney's teaching that I cleared my schedule and agreed to go.

It was a fascinating week. We started with *pranayama* every day, and even though it was gentle, the practice affected me in a way that felt uncomfortable but important. We continued learning about the health of the spine and the joints, and how yoga sequencing and alignment directly affect their longevity and ease. In the evening, he'd host activities, such as "Ask Rodney," a question-and-answer session. He hosted movies, discussions, even line dancing. Heidi and I didn't attend the evening gatherings and were amused at how much attention Rodney seemed to need from his students.

On the last day of the workshop, I was lying in *shavasana* and started to cry. It was unlike me to show emotion in public, and yet my tears soon turned into sobs. I had no idea why I was crying, just that something inside me had broken open. I knew that sometimes in yoga practice, our bodies tune in to things that our minds may not be ready to admit or deal with. I felt Rodney walk over and stand next to me, and I calmed down. Not a word had passed between us all week—I had taken copious notes but hadn't wanted to give him the satisfaction of getting a question from me. After *shavasana*, students started asking questions about the class, completely avoiding the elephant in the room. Finally, one person raised his hand. "What do you do when a student cries during *shavasana*?"

Rodney answered, "You leave them alone. You realize that he or she is probably the strongest and most honest person in the room. And you ask yourself, 'Why aren't we all crying?'" I was befuddled. He hadn't left me alone. He had come over to comfort me. I blurted out my first words of the week. "It was me who was crying, Rodney. And you came over and stood by me."

He looked surprised. "I'm sorry. I don't know what you're talking about. I never left my seat right here at the front of the room." I felt like my breath had been knocked out of me. I was totally confused. If he hadn't come and stood near me, then what had happened? I had no doubt that I had felt an undeniable energetic connection between us.

At the end of the workshop, Rodney gave all the students his email address and asked us to write to him if we had any questions. I thought that was odd—no other famous teachers had ever offered their email address so freely—but I took the information down and noticed that I had a lump in my throat while I was writing.

I waited a week and spent a lot of time formulating a smart and dispassionate question. Then I sent Rodney an email, reintroducing myself in case he didn't remember me, and asked him about the positioning of the pelvis in closed twists. He replied within hours and signed off with the words "I miss you." I was tingling from head to toe. Part of me was disgusted that he would say he missed me; he was probably coming on to me as rumor had it he did with many women, but another part of me was titillated and flattered that he remembered me.

We began emailing. I knew it was wrong. We were both married, with children. I told myself I needed—and wanted—to continue to study with Rodney. I convinced myself I owed it to my students to continue my education. I vowed I wouldn't cross any lines.

Over the next year, I made my way to almost every one of Rodney's workshops. He was an engineer of the human body, and I learned an enormous amount about the architecture and intricacies of the poses, which Rodney made illuminating and practical. I took the teaching back to my students and teachers, upping the game at Yoga Shanti. I still taught a Jivamukti-syle class with rock and roll music, but I became obsessed with sequencing for the nervous system and the health of the spine. I felt like I was doing graduate work, getting the education in a subject that I was passionate about.

Still, I was wary. Rodney had a reputation with the ladies—and I was determined not to become one of them. One evening at the end of a weeklong training in Nashville, I decided to go to the closing party. Over the years, I had been studying shiatsu with a man named Ohashi, and was interested in the energy meridians of the body. Rodney and I were sitting together, talking, and I reached over and put my thumb on the shiatsu point between his eyebrows called *do in*. Hindu culture says this is where the soul appears, and people adorn the spot with a *bindi*, the red dot I had seen in India. In shiatsu, the spot is more related to headaches and nasal congestion, so I'm not sure why I chose it. But the second I put my thumb between Rodney's eyebrows, we both felt an inexplicable charge.

That evening, I told him that I had no desire to sleep with him, but that I would like to spend twelve hours talking with him about yoga and life. I was staying with another student, and as we were leaving the party, Rodney asked if we'd give him a ride to his host's house. He was sitting in the backseat, and as we drove, he reached over and took hold of my hand. The three of us sat in the car in his host's driveway and talked into the wee hours of the morning.

We started a relationship. I'm not proud of it, and I truly regret that we hurt people in our lives. I tried not to see Rodney, but it didn't work. I did, in fact, become one of "those women," and I was riddled with guilt. Robin and Rodney's wife were good people. They didn't deserve our lies or the ensuing pain.

In 2003, almost a year after we began an affair, Rodney told me that he and his family were going to Bali for the summer. I thought this was the perfect opportunity to see if our marriages were salvageable. There would be no temptation as we would be ten thousand miles apart. I asked him to try to reconcile with his wife. I would do the same with Robin. I asked him not to call or write during the two months that he would be away. "If you do," I told him, "I won't respond."

Six days later, Rodney sent me an email. I was happy to receive it, but I didn't write back. Several days later, the telephone rang at 3:00 a.m. so I answered it, thinking my sister, Peggy, was calling with bad news. My father had fallen off his roof earlier that day while doing repairs and had been admitted to intensive care at the local hospital with a broken shoulder, broken ribs, and a punctured lung. But it was Rodney on the phone. He told me he couldn't live without me, that he had told his wife everything, and that he wanted to marry me: "I jumped, Colleen. Are you there to catch me?"

"No," I replied. "If you decide to leave your wife, it's for your own reasons." When I got back into bed, Robin asked who had called. I couldn't lie anymore. I told him everything. It was a night of utter devastation. We went through several months of turmoil, tears, and therapy, but there was no reconciliation to be had. Robin moved out, and a few months later, Rodney moved in.

The news rocked the yoga world, and the tabloids had a field day. We heard all the snickers as we fell off the pedestals people had put us on. The price of our relationship was high. I understand the urge to gossip and judge. I also understand the damage it causes. There's nothing about gossip that benefits the world. This was a huge lesson for me. Buddhists recommend asking four questions before you speak: Is it true? Is it kind? Is it necessary? And, lastly, does it improve on silence?

The fact that Rodney had been my teacher brought up a lot of discussion about the ethics of teacher-student relationships. I understand this inquiry and have thought long and hard about it myself. I don't have a hard-and-fast answer. Sometimes two people aren't on equal footing, and sometimes they are. I didn't feel there was a hierarchy of power between Rodney and me. We simply fell passionately and undeniably in love. The problem was that we were married to other people, and we both had children.

While Rodney was in the process of moving in, he said he wanted to go to Indiana with me for Christmas. I thought it was too soon, but he insisted. Rachel and I had been there for a few days when he showed up. At one point, all five of my very tall brothers were sitting around the kitchen table, and Mom pulled Rodney aside and pointed to them. "Look," she said. "That's a lot of brawn in there. You better not break my daughter's heart."

My family liked Rodney immediately. One night, we went to a local bar. As we were walking through the door, without saying a word, my brothers formed a protective phalanx around him. They weren't sure how the locals would react to someone who was Asian American, and felt a need to protect him. I knew he had been accepted.

Rodney is a talker. All his friends and students know it and love him for it. He can talk happily for hours. But from the beginning, he was also curious about what I had to say. And he listened. It was a new experience for me. Someone was genuinely interested in what I thought. Our backgrounds were similar, so it felt like we were cut from similar cloth: He wasn't from a privileged family. His father had been a colonel in the US Air Force, and his mother a stay-at-home mom. Rodney dropped out of college, just as I had. Our similarities went back to our forebears, the Chinese and Irish immigrants who came over and worked building the railroads. We found we had the same work ethic and spoke a similar language in every way.

So the long, arduous road toward divorce and the blending of families began. Even though I pride myself on being an expert yoga sequencer, I did a lousy job of sequencing these transitional events. Poor sequencing hurts people, and this was no exception. I wish I had split up with Robin before taking up with Rodney. I wish I had told Rachel the truth, before she found out on her own. Rodney had to deal with his own challenges. He left everything—his family, his friends, his yoga studio in Oakland, and his community—to be with me. He said doing anything else would have been a lie.

Not long after he came east, his wife, Donna, asked me to fly to California to see her. I did, and we went for a long walk. She said that she could see what Rodney and I had together, and she knew that she and Rodney hadn't had the same thing. She wanted me to know she didn't think badly of me, and she was giving her children full permission to love me. I was so overcome by her generosity and grace I wanted to marry her instead of Rodney.

Every family member dealt with seismic shifts. Rachel was just turning eight. Shortly after Rodney moved in, we were walking down the street in Sag Harbor when she insisted on holding both my hands so that I wouldn't be able to hold his. Before long, though, Rachel and Rodney's kids—Evan, Adesha, and JoJo—became a family. They bonded early, and strongly, which made the transition less traumatic.

My biggest regret to this day is having lied to Rachel. I told her Rodney was a friend who would be staying with us for a while, sleeping downstairs. Then one day she caught us kissing. I had broken her trust. Nothing devastated me as much as this. I conveniently thought I was protecting her, but in fact I created more damage.

Our first few years together were intense. There was no doubt Rodney and I loved each other, but was that enough? One day we drove out to a hotel in Montauk for a romantic night. I had gotten a sexy nightie for the occasion and went into the bathroom to put it on. When I came out, I found Rodney glued to the television, watching a ski race in the Winter Olympics, which he loves. I cleared my throat, but he barely looked up. "I'll be right there, just let me see the end of this race," he said.

I was beyond insulted. We fought all night and headed home first thing in the morning. I was still furious when we drove into our driveway. Like a crazy woman, I proceeded to throw every one of his belongings into the front yard. "Go back to California," I ordered. We argued until two o'clock that afternoon, at which point we were sitting on the bench in front of the house, exhausted, looking at all his stuff still on the lawn. I started laughing. He looked at me, and then he started laughing. Before long, we were both in hysterics. We cleaned up the yard. It felt like the sky had cleared after a hellacious storm. We blamed the fight on the fact that we were in the middle of a juice cleanse and were cranky. We abandoned the cleanse, and Rodney stayed.

Finding balance in who we were as a couple, as teachers, as coparents, and as part of our community took time and negotiation. We felt as if we were under a microscope, with inquiring eyes watching intently as we tried to figure out the dynamics of our new life. Many people thought we wouldn't last. We weren't sure either.

Balance is a key concept in yoga, whether it's trying to hold a difficult posture like Warrior III—where you suspend yourself in midair like Superwoman while balancing on one leg—or just noticing your body's subtle shifts while standing in Mountain Pose. Yogis are trying to find internal balance so that they won't be tossed around by changing currents. The Ayurvedic doctor Robert Svoboda says students often practice the kind of yoga they're good at, rather than what will bring them balance. He notes that those students who are practicing vinyasa should probably be doing restorative yoga, and those doing restorative should probably be practicing a more active and heat-inducing form of asana. But not many of us are willing to break out of our comfort zone in order to find balance.

Do Rodney and I balance each other? In many ways, we're very similar; we have the same priorities and values. In other ways, we're polar opposites. Physically, we couldn't be more different. He is thick, solid, and close to the ground. He's practical and of the earth. He was a ballet dancer before he discovered yoga. His approach to yoga is all about the engineering, architecture, and function of the body.

I'm the opposite. I used to long to be lost in space and travel to altered states. When we first started meditating together, I would ask Rodney, "Why are you sitting so rigidly? You look like you're posing for *Yoga Journal*." He, on the other hand, would get scared when I would float away in meditation. He said he could feel me leaving my body, and suddenly there was nobody there.

You could say Rodney ties me to earth, and I show him flight into the unknown. His understanding of the mechanics of the body was a missing link for me both personally and in my yoga teaching. For a kite to fly, it needs a tether. Rodney is my tether. He teaches me form, and I teach him formlessness. He shows me a practical, intelligent relationship to the earth, and I lure him into the element of mystery through devotion, chanting, and meditation. We're all searching for balance. But balance isn't a set point or destination; it's a constant play between opposites. In our early days, the energy and passion Rodney and I felt for each other was overwhelming. It ran wild and frequently hurt others. We needed to find balance.

✦ ✦ ✦

The fourth *yama*, or ethical precept of yoga, is called *brahmacharya*, which is translated as celibacy, containment, monogamy, or not misusing sexual energy. The sexual drive is a force that can cause a lot of imbalance if it's not used wisely.

I hadn't joined Mother Teresa's Missionaries of Charity, because a life of celibacy would have been a lie for me. I wasn't willing to take that vow as a yogi. But after seeing the chaos Rodney and I caused by not having proper energetic boundaries, I wanted—and needed—to find orientation, containment, and peace of mind. *Brahmacharya* is important for a yoga practice; it helps create steadiness of the mind. Rodney and I find that stability in our monogamous commitment. Our sexual energy is reserved for each other, and it feels honest, contained, and natural. It is the closest we will probably get to *brahmacharya*. As a result, we have more energy to focus on what is important to us—our family, yoga, and service.

The Sutras say that if you can practice one of the *yamas* or *niyamas* fully, the others fall into place. It also follows that if one is off balance, the others will be as well. That was our situation, but after the upheaval, we can see the truth (*satya*) and contentment (*santosha*) that come from nonharming (*ahimsa*) via containment (*brahmacharya*). With monogamy there is less distraction from sexual urges, and the mind can become clearer. We are still maneuvering toward balance, but the dance is becoming more subtle and intimate.

Rodney and I have become each other's teachers. When we got married, a friend told us that we were brave because we hold mirrors up to each other every day—and it's hard to see yourself reflected back all the time. We decided to teach in tandem so we could spend more time together. Initially, it was awkward. We would get angry at each other if one person went on too long, or didn't stick to the sequence we had planned, or didn't make the right transition from what the other person had taught. We figured it out through a lot of negotiation, practice, push, and pull. There are still times when Rodney talks too much and I go over my time limit, but we don't get as rattled. The drama has lessened.

A normal day is when Rodney wakes me up; I'm a little grumpy because I want more sleep. But I know consistency of practice is important. So I drag myself out of bed and into our yoga room where we sit facing each other for *pranayama* practice. Rodney then goes down to the kitchen and makes coffee for himself and tea for me. He brings my tea to our yoga room, and he goes back to the kitchen, where he keeps his mat. I stay and do my practice, and plan the sequences for the day's class; he does the same in the kitchen. (We tried practicing together, but he'd start talking and I couldn't concentrate. After much deliberation, we decided we were adult enough to practice in different rooms.) Most of the time, I fall into a zone and lose track of time. Rodney always knows what time it is and will yell up to me that we're late for class. Most days, one or both of us are teaching; the one who's not teaching always attends the other's class. We have only missed a handful of each other's classes during the last twelve years.

On the rare occasions we aren't teaching, we sit at the kitchen table or in our backyard, drinking coffee and tea and discussing whether the spread of the pinky toe creates more of an inhalation or an exhalation. We spend practically all day every day together, and people constantly ask us how we do it. My answer is we like to be together. My parents wished they could be together all the time. Rodney and I arrange our lives so it's possible.

Fortunately, our families have blended as seamlessly as our teaching. When we got married in Las Vegas in 2006, we invited our immediate families, which came to about eighty people, between siblings, parents, and nieces and nephews. From the moment our two clans met, they melded into one. It was the most integrated and fun gathering I have ever been a part of.

It has now been more than a decade since Rodney moved in, and we continue to navigate the intimacies of our love by exploring the delicate balance of life together. Thankfully, our bullfight has become a wonderful pas de deux.

Yoga Sequence: Finding Balance

Part of Rodney's and my navigation has been about negotiating the classroom together.

We set ground rules. For instance, I lead the students in opening meditation and introduce the theme for the class. If we are doing a backbend class, for example, I talk about what supports the lift of the chest. Rodney then talks for a few minutes about the dos or don'ts of the asana practice we are teaching and introduces a philosophical element.

In this sequence we are incorporating all categories of poses in an attempt to find balance between forward bends and backbends, closed twists and open twists, inhalation and exhalation, internal rotation and external rotation—all of which are the balance of downward wind (*apana*) and upward wind (*prana*). We practice the subtlety of relationships by keeping the recessive action alive while engaged in the dominant action, for instance, maintaining the magic of the backbend while in the forward bend and the magic of the forward bend while in the backbend. Each person has his or her own preferences. Rodney favors backbends; left to his own devices that's what he would practice. Backbends are energizing. It's not uncommon for extroverts and coffee drinkers to like backbends. Backbends elicit more of an inhalation; inhalations are enlivening and build more heat. My own preference is forward bends, which are calming and cooling, and turn one inward. Because forward bends focus on the exhalation, which is more relaxing, introverted herbal tea drinkers like me tend to be drawn to them. The point is, though, that if I did only forward bends and Rodney did only backbends, we wouldn't be as likely to find balance. You could say this sequence is the perfect combination of coffee and chamomile tea.

Most Eastern modalities aim for the equanimity that lies somewhere between male and female, yin and yang, dark and light. One of the common translations of *hatha* is "sun and moon." So hatha yoga involves the heat of the sun coupled with the coolness of the moon. Hopefully, this practice will leave you with a residue of both, which creates equanimity.

Meditation (dhyana). Sit on a folded blanket with your left shin crossed in front of your right. Notice the space in your torso. Does it feel like a spacious chapel with a high dome or does it feel like a dilapidated house? Do you feel you are being pulled in one direction or the other? What in your body is distracting you? Notice that putting the other shin in front will change the internal shape and space of your body. Now cross your right shin in front of your left and notice the difference. Stay and watch for 1 minute.

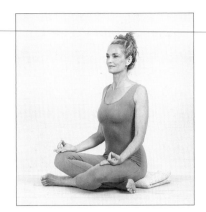

Meditation

Reclining Big Toe Pose (supta padangushthasana). To prepare for standing poses, place a strap around the ball of your right foot and lift your leg to the ceiling, extending your left leg along the floor (a). Stay for 5 breaths. Then hold the strap with your right hand and open your right leg out to the side for another 5 breaths (b). Switch sides. (If your hamstrings are tight, lengthen the strap.) Come to sit in Easy Pose, right shin in front of left.

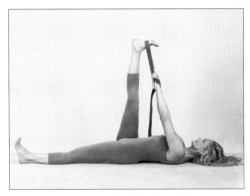

Reclining Big Toe Pose (a)

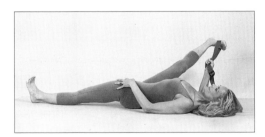

Reclining Big Toe Pose Variation (b)

Easy Pose with Side Bend and Backbend (sukhasana variation). Take your right hand to the floor about 1½ feet from your hips, extend your left arm into the air, and side bend to the right. Stay for 5 breaths (a). Inhale, lift up. Place the outside of your left wrist to the outside of your right knee and turn to the right for 5 breaths (b). Then drop your left shoulder to your left knee and swing your right arm up and over your right ear. Turn your chest to the ceiling as you lean into a slight backbend for 5 breaths (c). This lateral twist opens the side of the torso in preparation for backbends. Change sides and repeat the three poses with the left shin in front, twisting to the left. Then step back to Downward-Facing Dog.

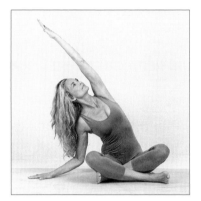
Easy Pose with Side Bend (a)

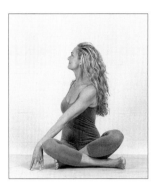
Easy Pose with Twist (b)

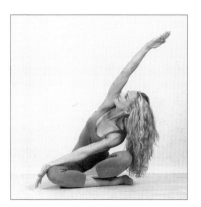
Easy Pose with Twist and Backbend (c)

Downward-Facing Dog with Side Bend (adho mukha shvanasana). Bend your right knee and pull it to the left, opening the left side of your body. Your weight shifts to your right hand and left foot. Hold for 5 breaths. Change sides and repeat, holding for 5 breaths. Walk your feet forward between your hands and come to Mountain Pose.

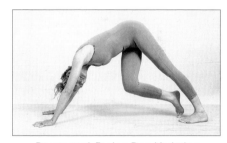
Downward-Facing Dog Variation

Volcano Pose Variation (urdhva hastasana). Standing with your feet hip-width apart, grip your left wrist with your right hand and stretch laterally to the right, leaning into a slight backbend. Hold for 5 breaths and repeat on the other side. Then take a 3½-foot step open to the right.

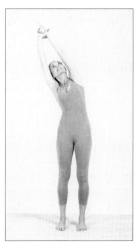
Volcano Pose Variation

Triangle Pose (trikonasana). Inhale as you lift your arms parallel to the floor and align your feet below your hands. Turn the left foot in slightly and the right foot out 90 degrees. Inhale into the foundation of your legs, then exhale and lower your right hand to a block behind your right foot (a). Reach your left arm to the ceiling, lengthening both sides of your torso evenly. Ground your back heel strongly to turn your chest toward the ceiling as you lean back on your shoulder blades. Hold for 5 breaths, then press your left foot into the floor strongly to stand up. Change sides and repeat. Step your feet together and return to **Mountain Pose** (b). Inhale, reach your arms up (c), exhale, and fold forward to **Standing Forward Bend** (d). Inhale and look forward, and exhale and step back to **Downward-Facing Dog** (e) before lowering down to your knees.

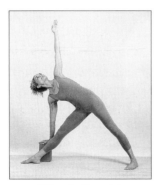

Triangle Pose (a)

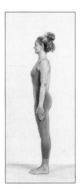

Mountain Pose (b)

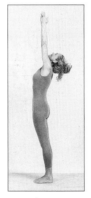

Arms Overhead (c)

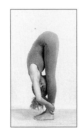

Standing Forward Bend (d)

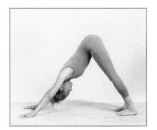

Downward-Facing Dog (e)

Gate Pose (parighasana). Kneeling at the center of your mat, turn sideways and extend your right heel out to the right in line with your left knee until your leg is straight. Slide your right hand down your right leg and reach your left arm up and overhead to stretch sideways with a hint of a backbend. Hold for 5 breaths, then change sides and repeat. Then sit in Staff Pose.

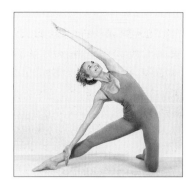

Gate Pose

Revolved Bent-Knee Seated Forward Bend (parivritta janu shirshasana). Bend your left knee and drop it to the left, then widen the thighs to more than 90 degrees. Drop your right elbow to the inside of the right leg and take your left hand behind your head to create support for your head as you turn toward the ceiling. Stay for 5 breaths (a). Then extend your left arm over your ear and lengthen your waist and arch your torso into a slight backbend (b). Hold for 5 breaths and repeat both variations on the other side. Return to Staff, cross your shins, step back to Downward-Facing Dog, then lower down onto your belly.

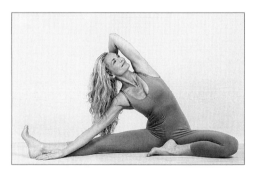

Revolved Bent-Knee Seated Forward Bend (a)

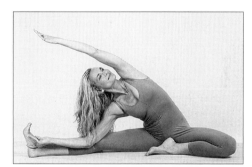

Revolved Bent-Knee Seated Forward Bend (b)

Cobra Pose (bhujangasana). Bend your elbows and press your palms to the floor alongside your chest, fingers pointing toward the front of your mat. Pull your chest forward into **Cobra Preparation** (a), creating a long waist. Lower down and repeat. Stay for 2 breaths each time. Slowly straighten your arms into Cobra, taking care not to hunch your shoulders. Repeat. Stay for 2 breaths each time (b). Exhale to release, and press back to **Downward-Facing Dog** (c).

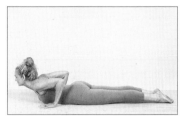
Cobra Preparation (a)

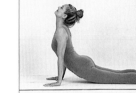
Cobra Pose (b)

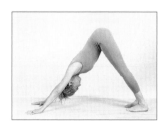
Downward Dog (c)

Side Plank Variation (vasishthasana variation). Shift onto the outside of your right foot, stack the left leg on top, and swing up onto your straight right arm. Step your top foot behind the bottom foot and lift your top arm up and back on a diagonal. Press your left foot strongly into the floor to lift the hips higher. Open the entire front of your torso into a backbend; hold for 5 breaths. Repeat on the other side. Then lie down on your belly.

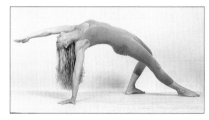
Side Plank Variation

Bow Pose (dhanurasana). Bend your knees and hold your ankles. Lift your thighs away from the floor and move your chest forward and up. Keep your lower ribs on the floor as you lift your legs higher. Hold for 3 breaths. After the asymmetry of open backbend twists, these symmetrical backbends set the sacrum evenly. Repeat, then roll over onto your back.

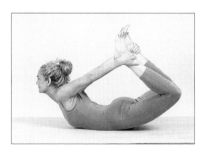
Bow Pose

Supported Bridge (setu bandha). Bend your knees and place your feet on the floor, hip distance apart, heels near the buttocks. Lift your hips and slide a block under your sacrum at the highest height that is comfortable. Stay for 20 breaths. Lift your hips, slide the block out, and lower down.

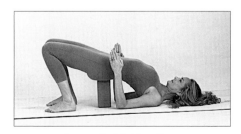
Supported Bridge Pose

Constructive Rest. Drop your knees together. Put your hands on your belly and enjoy watching 5 cycles of breath.

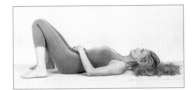

Constructive Rest

Reclining Big Toe Pose (supta padangushthasana). We revisit this neutral pose, allowing the spinal disks to absorb fluid and re-center themselves before moving into the closed twists and forward bends. Place a strap around the ball of your right foot and straighten your leg to the ceiling for 5 breaths (a). Switch sides. Then repeat the pose with your right leg, but this time move the strap to your left hand and press your right thumb deeply into your hip crease as you cross your leg 2 inches to the left. Hold for 5 breaths, return your leg to center, and exhale as you lift your head and chest toward your knee in a sit-up variation (b). Hold for 3 breaths. Release, repeat with your left leg, and roll to your side to sit up in Staff.

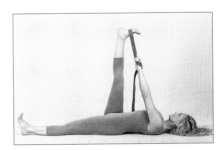

Reclining Big Toe Pose (a)

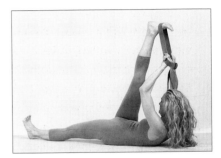

Reclining Big Toe Pose Variation (b)

Bent-Knee Seated Twist (marichyasana III). Bend your left knee and press your foot to the floor, heel as close to your sit bone as possible. Turn to the left and hug your left knee with your right arm for 5 breaths (a). Repeat to the right. Notice that the lower back is in more of a forward bend than in the open twists. Push forward into a **Squat** (b). Lift your hips into a Standing Forward Bend.

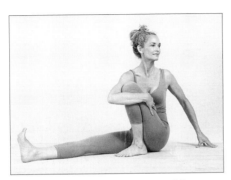

Bent-Knee Seated Twist (a)

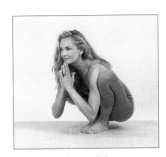

Squat (b)

Standing Forward Bend (uttanasana). Keep your legs engaged as you grab your ankles and pull them up toward the pelvis as you draw your head down toward the floor. Stay for 5 breaths.

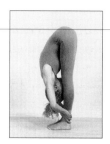

Standing Forward Bend

Revolved Side Angle Pose Variation (parivritta parshva-konasana variation). Step your right foot back to a lunge, come onto your right fingertips, press your left thumb into your outer left hip crease, and turn your torso to the left. Reach through your back leg strongly. Stay for 5 breaths. Step the back foot to the front of the mat and repeat on the other side.

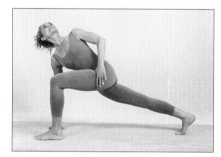

Revolved Side Angle Pose Variation

Revolved Side Angle Pose Variation (parivritta parshvakona-sana variation). Step your right foot back and place the knee on the floor. Turn to the left and place your right elbow on the outside of the left knee, make a fist with your right hand, and wrap the left hand around it. Hold for 5 breaths. Then step the back foot forward and repeat on other side for 5 breaths. Step forward and lift to stand at the front of your mat.

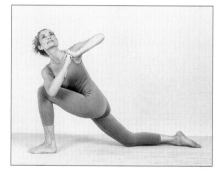

Revolved Side Angle Pose Variation

Flying Up Lock Mountain with Lion, Belly, and Throat Valves Applied (tadasana with simhasana, uddi-yana, and jalandhara bandha). Starting in Mountain, bend your knees slightly, place your hands on your thighs, inhale through your nose, then exhale energetically through your wide-open mouth, stretching your tongue out as far as possible (a). When your exhalation is complete, soften your knees, retract your tongue, drop your chin to your chest, and press your hands to your thighs to straighten your arms. Pull your belly toward your spine (b). Hold very briefly, then relax your belly, inhale, and come to standing. Repeat 3 times. If you feel lightheaded, stop. Always take a few normal breaths in between repetitions while feeling your feet and focusing on something that is not moving.

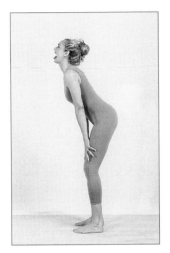

Mountain Pose with Lion (a)

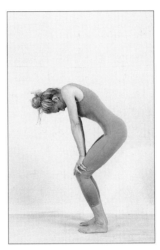

Mountain Pose with Lion, Belly, and Throat Valves Applied (b)

Intense Side Stretch (parshvottanasana). Step your right foot out to the right, then parallel your feet and bring your palms together between your shoulder blades or hold opposite elbows behind your back. Turn your left foot in 45 degrees and your right foot out 90 degrees, squaring your torso over your right leg. Inhale, lift your chest, and from the strength of your back leg, forward bend over the right leg for 5 breaths. Inhale to lift up, and repeat to the left. To finish, bring your feet parallel to each other.

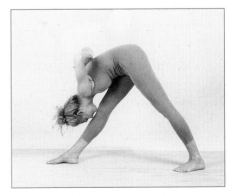

Intense Side Stretch

Revolved Triangle (parivritta trikonasana). With your hands on your hips, turn your left foot in 45 degrees and your right foot out 90 degrees, squaring your torso over your right leg. Raise your chest and lift your left arm up alongside your ear, then exhale as you take the left hand to a block on the outside of the right foot and extend your right arm up toward the ceiling (a). Hold for 5 breaths. Inhale, come up, and change sides. Turn your feet parallel and walk your feet together. Come to stand at the front of your mat. Inhale your arms up (b); exhale and fold forward (c); inhale, bend your knees, and look forward (d); then walk back to **Downward-Facing Dog** (e). Take your knees to the floor, cross your shins, and sit down behind your feet and extend your legs to **Staff Pose** (f).

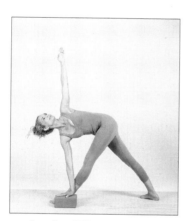

Revolved Triangle Pose (a)

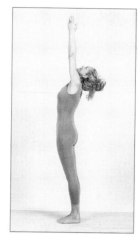

Arms Up (b)

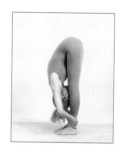

Standing Forward Bend (c)

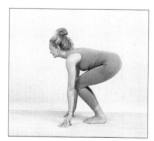

Bent-Knees Look Forward (d)

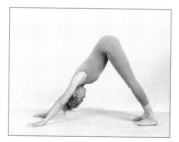

Downward-Facing Dog (e)

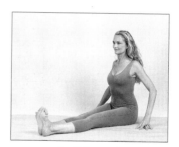

Staff Pose (f)

Wide-Legged Seated Forward Bend (upavishtha konasana). Open your legs as wide as you can and press them firmly down into the floor, reaching through the heels. Come forward any amount and support yourself with your arms, however is comfortable. Hold for 8 breaths and sit up with your hands behind you.

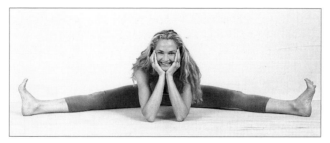

Wide-Legged Seated Forward Bend

Bound Angle (baddha konasana). Bend your knees and bring the soles of your feet together, then hold your big toes and come forward with a long waist (a). Hold for 5 breaths. Inhale, lift your torso, and stretch your legs to **Staff Pose** (b).

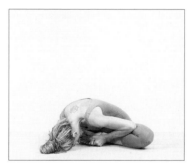

Bound Angle Pose (a)

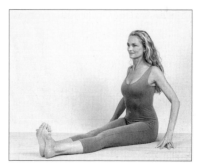

Staff Pose (b)

Seated Forward Bend (pashchimottanasana). Exhale and fold forward. Forward bends can be the most rejuvenating of all the poses, so make sure you don't strain and that your breath is smooth. Hold for 10 breaths.

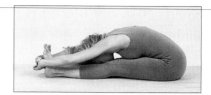

Seated Forward Bend

Meditation and Breath Expansion *(dhyana, pranayama).* Sit on a folded blanket. Feel the breath move your ribcage from front to back. As you exhale, keep the expanse of the ribcage. Repeat for 5 breaths. Then take 5 normal breaths. Now direct your inhalations so they spread your ribcage from side to side for 5 breaths. Come back to 5 normal breaths. Next, breathe so that the inhale lengthens the spine and the exhale slightly shortens it; repeat for 5 breaths. Come back to normal breathing and let the breath dance in the expanse of your torso while you watch it without manipulation for 1 minute.

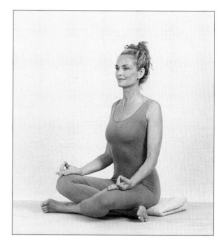

Meditation

Our next experiment in balanced breathing is a *pranayama* practice called **Alternate Nostril Breathing (nadi shodana).** Take your right hand to your face with a relaxed hand, inhale through both nostrils, then block the left nostril with your ring finger and exhale through the right nostril. Inhale through the right nostril and exhale through the left as you block the right nostril with your right thumb. Inhale left, exhale right. Do 8 cycles of Alternate Nostril Breathing. Take one more inhale through your right nostril, then release the hand and exhale naturally out of both nostrils as you float your head up to its normal position. Breathe naturally for 5 cycles of breath. Then sit quietly. For 5 minutes, observe this open chamber of the chest that can deal equitably with whatever life sends your way.

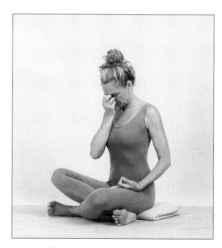

Alternate Nostril Breathing

Final Relaxation (shavasana). Strap your legs mid-thigh to keep your legs parallel. Place a bolster under your knees to release any strain on your back. Arrange your body evenly and comfortably. Remain alert and relaxed as you meditate on every cell of your body.

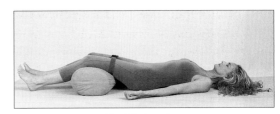

Final Relaxation

Early on in Rodney's and my relationship, I sent him Lucinda Williams's CD *Essence*. The title song became our song. It's about having to dig deep to find your essence. Yoga gives us the signposts that lead toward our essence and the tools to peel back the layers covering it up. The more we play to our habits, the further we stray from center, where many teachers say the true self resides. In yoga, we call this *sat guru*, or the guru that is always near. I often close my classes with the ritual Jivamukti chant: *Om bolo shri sat guru bhagavan qui,* which means "I bow down to the true teacher that dwells within." The class chants back an enthusiastic *Jai!* That means "Right on," or "Hallelujah!"

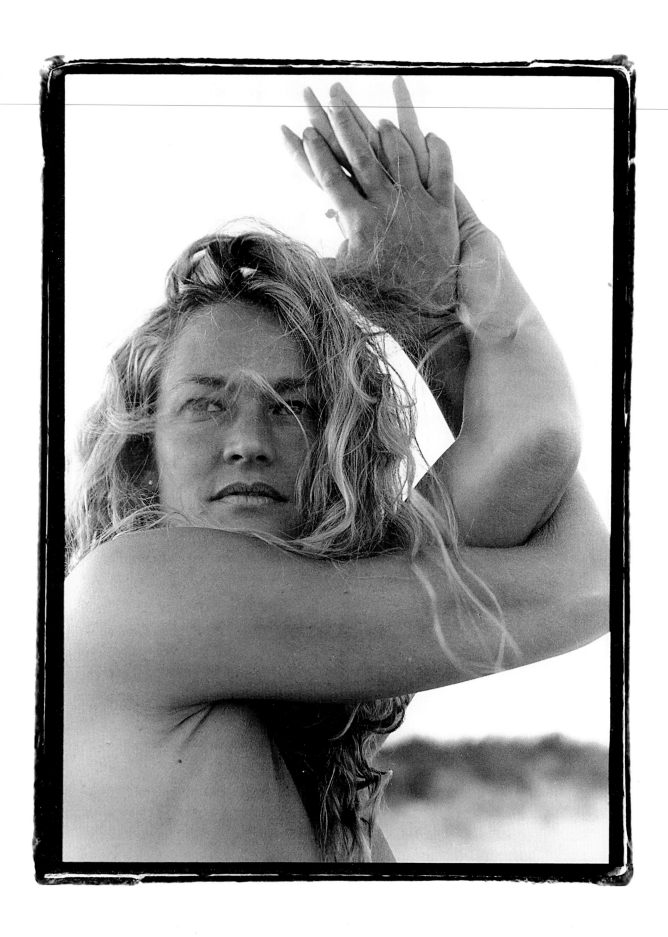

Chapter 13

WOMEN

Our deepest fear is not that we are inadequate. Our deepest fear is that we are powerful beyond measure. It is our light, not our darkness, that most frightens us. We ask ourselves, "Who am I to be brilliant, gorgeous, talented, fabulous?" Actually, who are you not to be?
—A Return to Love: Reflections on the Principles of
"A Course in Miracles," Marianne Williamson

All the women in my family start menopause early. At forty-two, I was deep in the throes of hot flashes and night sweats. I'm sure some people would have described me as cranky and emotionally erratic, but the truth is I just didn't feel like putting up with stuff I'd always put up with anymore. I spoke up, when previously I would have stayed quiet. Relationships that relied on my being the voiceless pretty girl came to an end—or changed radically. I don't think it was a coincidence that I fell in love with Rodney and left my marriage around the same time I began to go through menopause. By the time women get to menopausal age, we're generally less inclined to go along with the roles society has set forth for us. Our energetic currents are powerful at this age, which drives change. My friend, women's-health-and-wellness physician Christiane Northrup, calls this time "the lifting of the long hormonal veil." It can be both liberating and unsettling.

Menopause is a breakthrough, not a crisis or an illness. Rather than thinking of it as losing our fertility, our looks, and our purpose in the world, we need to recognize it as the time to step into our wisdom, to find our voices and our truth. There are more than 500 million postmenopausal women in the world—more than 50 million in the United States alone. I'd put money on the likelihood that many of us make major life changes at this juncture.

My shifts at midlife were all-inclusive. My sense of smell became much more acute, and smells that I used to love—perfumed moisturizers, scented candles—now turned my stomach. I craved cheese and eggs. Before menopause, my sex drive was associated with my ovulation cycle and would kick into high gear when my body was ripe for pregnancy. After menopause, sex became more about seduction, sensuality, and pleasure. Even my walk changed: Before menopause, I used to prance on my toes, like a puppy wanting to please its master. After, I walked heel to toe, and according to close friends and family, with a sort of swagger. I wasn't in such a hurry to please.

I cared less about what other people thought about me. And yet I found I needed the support of other women. When my marriage ended and my relationship with Rodney became public, my mom, sister, and dear friend Aida were my confidantes. As women, they could understand my aching heart.

Women need women. We need to be able to put down our burdens and fall apart, and we can do this with other women. When men aren't around, liberation takes place. Competition diminishes, and we feel supported in whatever we're going through.

Transformation occurs when women sit with one another for any length of time. Throughout history, we have done this—in sewing circles, menstrual huts, even on playgrounds. These days, we're so busy being superwomen we rarely make time for girlfriends. There's so much value in gathering to talk, laugh, and cry.

✦　✦　✦

Fifteen years ago, several of my female students asked me to lead an all-women's yoga retreat. I resisted. I was more comfortable with men, and I wasn't sure an all-women's week would be fruitful. I also felt insecure. The women asking me to lead the retreat were lawyers, doctors, politicians, newscasters, and Hollywood producers. I thought they were out of my league, but finally I agreed. What I found were women just like me, with the same hang-ups, who wanted to let down their defenses and feel relief from everyday demands.

Over the years, I've come to realize that woman-to-woman groups have immeasurable transformative potential. The process needs to be gradual, and requires trust. Most of us have been holding on to our "stuff"—the obstacles that keep us from expressing ourselves honestly and without apology—for a lifetime. Often we don't even know what it is that's keeping us stuck, because it is hidden so deeply in the body.

On the first afternoon of my now annual all-women's retreat in Mexico, forty or so women meet in a yoga room overlooking the water and sit in a big circle. I jokingly call it the "dreaded sharing circle." Dreaded as it may be, the circle is important. Each woman introduces herself and says where she's from and why she's there. Attendees have ranged from teenagers to octogenarians. The majority are middle-aged and are dealing with stresses of career changes, dying parents, dormant or fraying marriages, troubled kids, kids leaving home, and, for many, the seismic changes of menopause and aging. Some are trying to make sense of a life that has taken unexpected turns. Others are exhausted and need to reconnect to themselves and nature. Still others are facing big decisions and are looking for clarity. Some just want to do yoga with women, eat healthy food, and get a tan.

Most of these women get nervous about "sharing." Many have jobs that require public speaking, but when things get personal and real, they become very self-conscious. All of us spend the moments before we speak planning what we're going to say, then probably spend the rest of the time wishing we had said something else. But magic happens. By the time the last woman speaks, there's so much compassion in the room that the retreat has already been worthwhile.

Each retreat has a theme. Last year's was forgiveness. Previous retreats considered loneliness, trauma, secrets, even getting in touch with our perineums. I ask everyone to bring a journal in which to write for twenty minutes after each class. It's mandatory that all the participants attend every class—a total of five hours a day. The yoga room becomes a chamber of intimacy and release; the deeper we dig, the more vulnerable we become. If one person opts out, there's a palpable leak in the container. The combination of asana, *pranayama*, meditation, and journaling ignites a virtual sweat lodge that fuels us to search, reflect, and share. Many participants come year after year. We have supported one another through our worst times and our best.

Everyone hides traumas and secrets in different places. During the retreat, we systematically move through the body, using sequences to open targeted areas like the hips and the heart. After class, we write down what may have been buried in that area. As Rodney says, each of us has a place that's unbearable, where we don't want to go. In the safe haven of a women's retreat we can explore that place and find support through yoga and companionship. As memories and secrets are uncovered, emotions flow freely and possibilities of other ways of being surface.

One year a woman who is a rock star in her field ran out of the first class, sobbing. She walked straight into the ocean without breaking stride, tore off her shirt, and hurled it into the waves, screaming through her tears that she was throwing her shame away with her shirt; the ocean could have them both. She weighed more than two hundred pounds at the time, and she walked proudly, bare-breasted, out of the waves. Later, she shared that she had discovered the day before her departure that her husband was having an affair. It wasn't the first time. When she returned home, she turned her life around. She lost more than fifty pounds and left her husband. She was done being a victim and says now, "I'm working to find a way to be an honest parent and a compassionate ex-partner—and to forgive myself on days that grace is nowhere near."

Women often come to tears in the yoga room. If we can be honest while working deeply in our bodies, perhaps we can be honest in our speech. What good is the gift of language if what we're saying isn't true? We can feel it when someone is being real. It touches the centers of our being, and we are inspired to reveal ourselves.

◆　　◆　　◆

Voice has been my lifelong issue. I have given authority to men in many realms of my life. Watch any film that has a fashion model as a character: Everything that comes out of her mouth is dumb and superficial. Models are meant to be seen and not heard.

I played the role, but it never felt good. Growing up in a household full of smart boys made me tough, but it also made me think I had no business speaking because they had no interest in what I had to say. As recently as last year, the title of our family website was "Zello Bros." My sister brought it to my attention, and we rebelled. Now it says "Zello Bros. (and Sisters)." (Peggy and I are lobbying to get rid of the parentheses.)

Early in my teaching career, I realized that my life experience had given me some pretty valuable street smarts. In my classes, I spoke boldly on subjects I understood intimately from life itself. I chanted to Ganesh, the elephant-headed remover of obstacles, and just as Sharon and David had predicted, my off-key chanting inspired others to chant, even if they weren't in perfect pitch.

At national yoga conferences twenty years ago, the majority of teachers were men, while 90 percent of the practitioners were women. But men don't know the cycles of a woman's body or what brings relief to an aching uterus after a miscarriage. They don't know how it feels to menstruate, give birth, or go through menopause. They don't understand what a woman's heart feels like when it's betrayed. And women's shoulders, hips, knees, and ankles are structured differently.

Nature is round and sensuous; the alignment of the body and the flow of postural movements should embody these characteristics. By our very natures, women are more likely to tap into this perspective. A lightbulb went off for me when I took classes from Angela Farmer and Patricia Walden. Angela invited us to explore the fluidity and curvaceousness of the body in a circular, voluptuous way. She wasn't giving us angular and specific alignment points as a "one size fits all" class. It was feminine and sensual and taught from her body to ours. Patricia teaches from an intuitive perspective on women's specific emotional needs.

Today at national yoga conferences, the majority of participants are female, and the percentage of women instructors is more than 50 percent.

Menopause is a time for women to speak, not to shut down. As we get in touch with our internal power, we have much more to say. Dr. Christiane Northrup describes it this way: "As these hormone-driven changes affect the brain, they give a woman a sharper eye for inequity and injustice, and a voice that insists on speaking up about them. . . . They uncover hidden wisdom—and the courage to speak it. As the vision-obscuring veil created by reproductive hormones begins to lift, a woman's youthful fire and spirit are often rekindled, together with long-sublimated desires and creative drives. Midlife fuels those drives with a volcanic energy that demands an outlet."

Amen. The end of menses is a rite of passage, and we should celebrate it.

Yoga Sequence:
Trusting Our Intuition and Finding Our Voices

My classes and practice are no longer solely about range of motion or getting a good workout. My body guides my teaching, and I'm happy to say that, for the most part, I know how to listen. It's more sensitive and less forgiving now. When you're young, your body can withstand bad sequencing and daring gymnastics. Feedback comes more rapidly in a mature body. I used to cover up my intuitive impulse not to follow instructions—on and off the mat—for fear of looking stupid. Problems abound when we ignore the wisdom of the body.

The hormonal changes of menopause usually start about six years before menstruation ends and continue for several years after, so women spend about a tenth of their lives in perimenopause or menopause. As with all transitions, adjusting can be uncomfortable, with common symptoms like sweats, fatigue, fuzzy brain, anxiety, irritability, depression, and insomnia. And because our muscles lose some of their strength and speed, our joints can become unstable.

This sequence addresses these symptoms, giving women the opportunity to listen to the messages that underlie physical sensation. It's a restorative series that allows the nervous system to relax, but the practice also creates strength in the muscles and tone in the pelvic floor, which can lose firmness and elasticity. Restorative poses relieve fight-or-flight stressors while raising serotonin levels, which helps insomnia and stabilizes mood swings. And forward bends promote freedom and completion of the exhalation, which cultivates relaxation, a remedy for sleeplessness. Also included are poses to unlock your throat so your wisdom finds its voice.

Stepping out of competition and joining forces with other women can lead you into the next phase of life with freedom and clarity. So give yourself the time to step back, trust your intuition, observe your body and breath, discover (or rediscover) your voice, and let your practice nurture you.

Wide-Legged Standing Forward Bend (prasarita padottanasana). Stand at the front of your mat and step out 3 feet to the right. Take your hands to your hips, inhale, and lift your chest. Then exhale, fold forward, and rest your head on the floor (a) or on a block or two (b), depending on the height you need to make the head and neck comfortable. Keep your legs active. Stay for 3 minutes, then keep your head down as you walk your feet to hip distance apart.

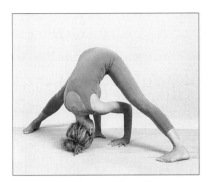

Wide-Legged Standing
Forward Bend (a)

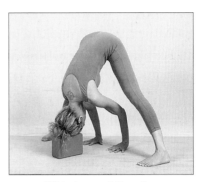

Wide-Legged Standing
Forward Bend with Block (b)

Standing Forward Bend with Blocks (uttanasana). Adapting the height of your blocks as necessary, rest the top of your head on blocks and stay for 3 minutes (a). Keep your head low as you turn toward the front of your mat and walk back to **Downward-Facing Dog** (b). Stay in the pose just long enough to determine where your head is so you can place a block under it. Position the block under your head, keeping your arms and legs straight and active (c). These postures bring fresh oxygenated blood and energy to the brain, which helps clear up fuzzy thinking. They also create strength in the large muscles of the legs and tone the pelvic floor. Stay for 2 minutes, then take your knees to the floor and get your bolster.

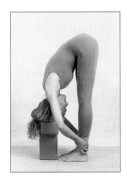

Standing Forward
Bend with Blocks (a)

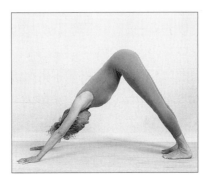

Downward-Facing Dog (b)

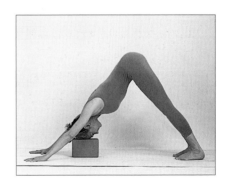

Downward-Facing Dog with Block (c)

Supported Child's Pose (balasana). Sit on your heels and spread your knees wide. Pull one end of the bolster into your pelvis, drape your body over it, and turn your head in one direction, then the other, for 1 minute per side (a). Very slowly come to sit on your heels. Take 3 breaths, then move to all fours, cross your shins, and sit down behind your feet. Straighten your legs to **Staff Pose** (b).

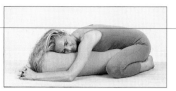

Supported Child's Pose (a)

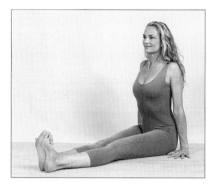

Staff Pose (b)

One-Legged Seated Forward Bend (janu sirsasana). Sit on a folded blanket, bend your left knee deeply, and open it out to a little more than a 90-degree angle with your left foot touching your left inner thigh (if possible). Place your bolster or a chair over your right leg and rest your forehead on the support as you fold forward for 2 minutes. Change legs and repeat. Restorative forward bends cool the head and allay anxiety and irritability. Inhale as you come up to sit on the edge of your blanket in Staff Pose.

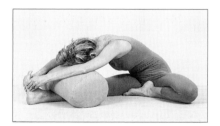

One-Legged Seated Forward Bend

Two-Legged Seated Forward Bend (pashchimottanasana). Adjust your bolster or chair so your forehead is easily supported as you fold forward. This pose turns you inward. Stay for 5 minutes.

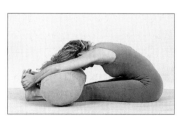

Two-Legged Seated Forward Bend

Supported Half Plow Pose (ardha halasana). Fold three blankets and place a chair 2 feet from the edge of the blankets. Lie down with your shoulders close to the edge and your head and most of your neck off the blankets. Swing your legs up and overhead, resting your toes on the seat of the chair and pressing your hands into your back, upper arms pressed against the blankets. (Don't let your elbows splay out.) Stay for 2 minutes. Come down slowly and slide off the blankets. This pose releases neck, back, and shoulder tension. Place your hands on your belly and watch 5 cycles of breath.

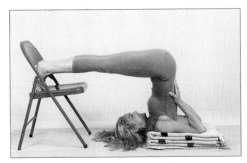

Supported Half Plow Pose

Supported Reclining Bound Angle Pose (supta baddha konasana). Place the bolster lengthwise along your mat and sit on a folded blanket in front of it. Take the soles of your feet together and spread your knees wide, supporting them with blocks. Lie back over the bolster and place another blanket under your head. If you feel too exposed, place a blanket over your pelvis. Stay for 5 minutes.

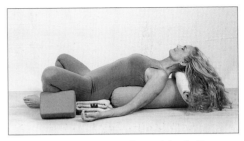

Supported Reclining Bound Angle Pose

Inverted Staff Pose (viparita dandasana). Position a chair on your mat about leg's distance from the wall, seat facing out. Place two blocks at medium height against the wall and set your bolster on the floor near the chair's front legs. Place a blanket on the chair seat and sit down, then thread your legs through the opening between the backrest and the seat. Place your feet on the blocks, knees slightly bent, and move your buttocks toward the wall until your sacrum rests on the back edge of the seat. Lower your torso and rest your shoulder blades on the front edge of the chair. Release your head back to the bolster (you may need a folded blanket on top) (a). Stay for 1 to 3 minutes with your arms stretched overhead or gripping the sides of the chair. This pose opens the throat and chest. Come up slowly by holding on to the sides of the chair and pressing your elbows into the seat, letting your head trail your torso. Then sit quietly, head bowed, for a few breaths. If the pose is too difficult, take **Fish Pose Variation** by placing a bolster under your shoulder blades; lie back and press your straight legs into the floor for 1 to 3 minutes (b).

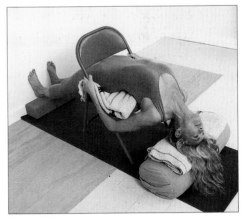

Inverted Staff Pose (a)

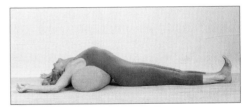

Fish Pose Variation (b)

Supported Legs Up the Wall Pose (viparita karani). Sit sideways against the wall; roll onto your back as you raise your legs up the wall. Bend your knees slightly, push into the wall with your feet to lift your pelvis, and place a block under your sacrum about 6 inches away from the wall so your sit bones dangle between the block and the wall. Rest your arms and hands on the floor, palms up, and stay for 3 minutes. This pose helps blood return to the heart, relieves tired legs, and improves digestion and circulation. In my opinion, it also improves sex drive.

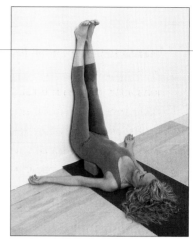

Supported Legs Up the Wall Pose

Final Relaxation (shavasana). Strap your legs mid-thigh and place a sandbag on the tops of your thighs. Place the bolster lengthwise along your mat and lie down on it, using a folded blanket for a pillow. Stay for 5 minutes.

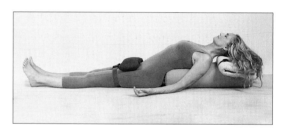

Final Relaxation

Meditation after Shitali Breath. Sit in a comfortable cross-legged position. Stick out your tongue, curl it, and sip an inhalation of breath through the cylinder you've created. If you cannot curl your tongue—it is genetic—stick it out and sip the air that way. Exhale through your nostrils. Practice 10 Shitali breaths, then sit with anything that arises for several minutes. This is a cooling breath and will give relief from the heat symptoms of menopause. The breath is a bridge between the body and the mind. Notice your body and what stories your mind is telling while you do this practice. Sit for 5 minutes.

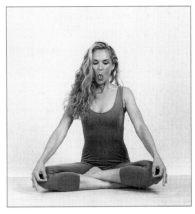

Meditation after Shitali Breath

Chant *Om mani padme hum* varying from a whisper to full voice and back to a whisper. The translation is "Hail to the jewel that sits in the seat of the lotus." Then sit in silence for another minute. You can decide where the seat of the lotus is for you, and know that you are uncovering a precious and unique jewel.

We have the power to change the way we view aging, but any shift in perspective needs to start from inside. Stagnation and deterioration are not age-specific. I've met as many stagnant twenty-year-olds as seventy-year-olds. Yoga helps us age with grace. By maintaining fluidity and mobility in body and mind, we're alive to the unfolding mystery and beauty of life. Yoga has taught me to stand aligned with truth and to use my voice to speak it. May this practice support you to do the same.

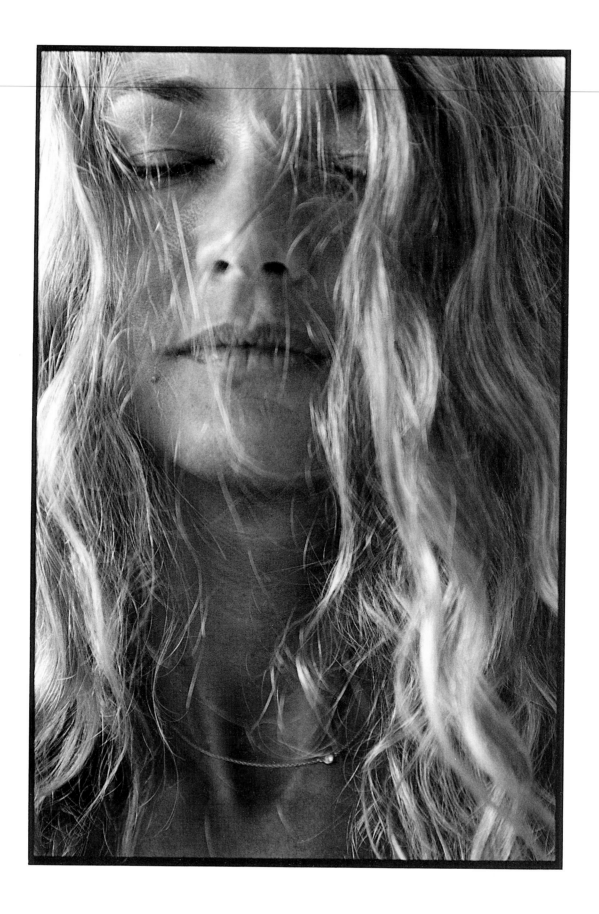

Chapter 14

PEACE

Student, tell me, what is God?
He is the breath inside the breath.
—"Breath," Kabir (tr. Robert Bly)

It's summer and Rachel is home from her first year at college. She has a job teaching at a local sailing camp. She has to be there at 8:00 a.m. At 7:00, I crawl into her bed to wake her up. I wrap my arms around her and breathe in the delicious smell of my daughter, whom I've missed so desperately for the past nine months. I'm holding her when I notice her chest is heaving. I pick my head up just enough to see her tears and the wet pillow. I can't ask her why she's crying because she won't tell me if I ask. So I hold her and let her cry.

Eventually, she tells me that she's been waking up in the mornings with a pit in her stomach. She feels guilty that either she's hurt someone, or didn't study enough, or has eaten too much junk food. I'm stunned, frozen, and broken. Have I passed on to Rachel the guilt gene that my mother passed to me? I thought I had successfully kept that from her, but I feel I've failed as a parent—again.

It seems like yesterday that I was walking around New York City with Rachel snuggled up to me in a baby carrier. I was floating with bliss, but also overcome with anxiety: *Who am I to be someone's mom?* My own mother, who was visiting at the time, told me, "It goes so fast, Colleen. Before you know it, she'll be off to college. That's when the really tough stuff starts—when you can't peek into her room anymore, hear her breathing, and know that she's safe." When we mothers worry about our kids, reason seems to fly out the window. Children can light up our hearts one minute and tear them apart the next. Parenting is like a yoga practice. It takes patience and discipline and dedication, it's full of ups and downs, and there is no end-game. Kids are the ultimate teachers.

The four sublime Buddhist attitudes are tailor-made for parents: We can greet happiness with loving-kindness (*Maitri*), unhappiness with compassion (*Karuna*), right behavior with joy and celebration (*Mudita*), and nonvirtuous behavior with equanimity (*Upeksha*). I try not to dwell too much on what I did or continue to do wrong or right as a parent, but it's difficult. If we don't find loving-kindness, compassion, joy, and equanimity, we suffer.

I haven't figured out how to take away Rachel's pain, whether it was from getting her bucket stolen in the sandbox or being bullied by girls in ninth grade. I was in Canada at a yoga conference when I got a call from her. I could barely make out what she was saying between her sobs, but she was asking me what was wrong with her. She wanted to know why the other girls would leave the table whenever she sat down with her lunch tray. The whole cafeteria could see them, and it humiliated her. She was being bullied and it broke my heart. Then one morning she came downstairs with her hair in a bun, wearing dangling earrings. She saw my surprise at this new look and said, "You know what, Mom? Nobody likes me anyway, so I can be whoever I want." Was she already digging around the yoga question: *Who am I?*

Rachel still hasn't completely forgiven me for leaving Robin and lying to her about Rodney, but, then again, I'm still working on forgiving myself. Jivamukti's cofounder Sharon Gannon used to say, "Inhale the word *let* and exhale the word *go*." Inhale, breathe in my guilt; exhale, breathe out forgiveness. Inhale, breathe in the meanness of the schoolgirl bullies; exhale, breathe out love for them.

It's a modern take on an ancient Buddhist meditation practice called *tonglen* in which we connect with suffering—our own and others'—through the breath. Breathe in suffering and pain and breathe out love and kindness. There are days, still, that I try to dedicate my practice to the mean girls who made Rachel's life miserable, but the intention gets stuck in my throat, and I switch the dedication to someone else before belting out my *oms*. By not forgiving them, I hurt myself, but I also need to be sincere in my dedications.

Clinging and aversion keep us from being in the present moment. I have heard, read, and felt this over and over. When I dropped Rachel off for her first day of preschool, my feeling of clinging was intense. No amount of concentrating on my breath or thinking about my feet connecting to the earth helped. I felt the same way when I dropped her off at college and walked down the dorm hallway without her. I wanted to run back and grab her and tell her not to grow up and leave me. But I kept walking, even though with each step the air got thicker and my breath less accessible. Inhale *let*; exhale *go*.

I have been studying and practicing yoga for the last twenty-eight years, learning how to avoid clinging to what is impermanent as gracefully as possible, and to focus on what doesn't change—call it the higher self, love, the soul, God, the divine, true teacher, essence, original nature, or the state of yoga—whatever you want. Intellectually, I get it, but when my baby girl leaves home and my mom dies, I am still in excruciating pain. These are the times when my practice saves my life. These are also the times when I feel most resistant to practicing. My advice is when you're feeling this way, drag yourself to class. If class is not an option, get on your mat and move or just lie in *shavasana*, and connect to your body and breath.

✦ ✦ ✦

On December 12, 2011, I got a call from my sister, Peggy. She sounded strangely direct and formal. "Colleen, it's about Mom. She's on her way to the hospital. We're not sure if she's going to make it."

It seemed impossible. My mom had just celebrated her eighty-first birthday. She had been Christmas shopping earlier that day and had texted me a couple of times about what she was getting the kids. Just that morning she had had breakfast with Peggy and had asked about the date she'd arranged for her (Peggy's husband of thirty-one years had died suddenly the year before). Peggy told her that the date had been wildly successful, and she was pretty sure she would marry this man. Mom knew it, too, and was at peace. All her babies were safe and in good places.

That afternoon, my dad heard her in the bedroom talking to a friend on the phone. When the chatter stopped suddenly, he went in to check on her. Mom was slumped in the chair, the phone on the floor. She had no pulse. He called 911, and the operator talked him through CPR. By the time the ambulance arrived, her heart had started beating again, but barely.

Earlier in the day, Rodney and I had been driving to the grocery store in Sag Harbor. A deer limped across the road in front of the car. One of its legs was broken and it looked like its spirit was leaving its body. That was hours before Peggy's call, but I'd turned to Rodney and said, "Mom's dying."

Rachel and I flew to Fort Wayne, Indiana, the next morning. The minute we walked into the hospital room, I saw the resignation in her eyes. I had the same helpless feeling I'd had as a girl, watching her cry over her lost trees, but now I had something with which to help her—and me. I put frankincense oil on my hands, crawled into bed with her, and held her head so she could see Rachel. They looked into each other's eyes while I gave her Reiki. I steadied my own breath. Mom's breath relaxed with mine. It was a precious, beautiful, and heart-wrenching moment.

Machines kept Mom alive for five more weeks. It was clear that she was done with her body and ready to shed it. The body is a gift given to us, only for a lifetime. When we die and the soul departs, the shell is left to be cremated or buried. My mom didn't have an easy life, but she lived a complete one. She gave birth to, nurtured, and adored seven children; she loved one man unreservedly; and she dedicated her life to her faith. On a cold morning in January, the doctors told my dad that her kidneys had shut down. He knelt at her bedside and kissed the love of his life for the last time.

We grow up knowing our mothers will leave us one day. I thought yoga had helped me with letting go, with understanding that everything changes and the most we can do is to be present. I thought my practice of dying a little every day—*shavasana*—was readying me for these bigger deaths. Why, then, did I feel so lost, lonely, sad, betrayed, and angry? I'd spent three decades being intimate with my body and breath through asana and *pranayama* practice, studying ideas of attachment and detachment in yoga philosophy. Still I was a puddle on the floor.

I'm grateful for the teaching of Roshi Joan Halifax. She says when dealing with death, we need to have a broad back of equanimity and a soft front of compassion. Instead of running away or numbing myself as I had done so often in my life, I did as Roshi Joan and Pema Chödrön counsel: I sat with the pain. I felt the gripping from my diaphragm all the way to my throat. I settled into my back body and tried to keep my front body soft to embrace what Pema calls the genuine heart of sadness. You touch it when you realize it is not just *your* pain, but *the* pain. That's how compassion and empathy can be born—understanding that sadness, anger, and brokenness are part of everyone's life. "There is a brokenness out of which comes the unbroken" is one of my favorite lines from Rashani Réa's poem.

Dad's grief at Mom's passing was as fervent as his devotion to her. As his unabashed and primal sobs shook the house, I thought of the story of the famous Indian guru whose son had died. His devotees showed up every day to find the guru crying and unable to give his dharma talk. Finally, one of the students asked, "Guruji, why is an enlightened man like you crying?" He replied, "I am crying because I am sad." There is nothing enlightened about not feeling. If you can't feel the fullness of any emotion, you're not fully alive.

✦   ✦   ✦

How do we experience peace when kids are leaving home, friends and parents are dying, health is failing, careers are changing, loved ones are hurting, countries are tearing themselves and one another apart with wars, and we're all exhausted? How do we live a life full of gratitude, love, and peace? It's even more important to find a tether to internal peace when things are falling apart. Peace is always there, deep within you. Sometimes the layers covering it up are thicker than at other times. It takes practice to get to peace in times of struggle. The more you practice, the more accessible it will be when your world is crumbling.

One of Rodney's and my favorite videos is of the Dalai Lama meditating. He's holding a small basket of what looks like chunky costume jewelry. When he loses his concentration, the basket of jewelry drops and the pieces scatter all over his lap and onto the floor. He opens his eyes, smiles, and picks up each piece one at a time, without frustration. He puts them all back in the basket and closes his eyes and returns to his meditation. This process repeats itself over twenty minutes. Here's the message: It's not about how many times you lose your focus and drop the jewelry. It's about picking up the pieces, and doing it over and over again with kindness toward yourself and others. A grip loosens. Things fall. A softening takes place.

Know you're enough. Just hearing Jason Isbell sing those words one day created in me an incredible sense of relaxation and comfort. I didn't know, or even care, what he was talking about. His singing, "Cover me up and know you're enough" was one of those aha moments, and since then, I use those words as my internal mantra over the diminishing refrain "less than."

For me, "know you're enough" answers yoga's core question, *Who am I?* It's these words that inspire me to be courageous on and off the mat. They make me feel I can do anything because I have nothing to lose or gain. I am already enough. I can stop struggling and simply see the person who spent a good part of her lifetime hiding behind feelings of inadequacy, fear, overcompensation, and perfectionism.

On one of the Dalai Lama's recent trips to the United States, he asked the audience what the main struggle was for individuals in the West. The answer was "low self-esteem." It took him awhile to even grasp the concept, which apparently doesn't exist in Tibetan culture. When he finally understood, his whole demeanor changed; he went from being jolly and conversational to being quiet and visibly sad.

Why do we fear we're not enough? What is it we're afraid of—that others will think less of us if we show them the truth? Fear causes alienation. You *are* enough. Knowing this for yourself may require a willingness to be uncomfortable as you dig through the rubbish to find the gem of the True Self. It's there. As the Indian mystic and poet Kabir wrote: "God is the breath within the breath." If *God* isn't the right word for you, try *love*. Love is the breath within the breath. If someone told you that what you had spent your whole life searching for was right under your nose, wouldn't it make sense to look there? We are already home, we just don't know it.

I've talked to many yogis over the years and asked them a simple question: "How has yoga affected your life?" One answer comes up consistently: that even though people have the same emotional triggers and reactions that they had before taking up yoga, their recovery time is much faster. It isn't that jealousy or anger ceases to exist when a button is pushed, but yogis can see the chain reaction and step back from it more quickly. Life becomes less exhausting, more enjoyable. This is one of the few promises I will make you.

✦ ✦ ✦

Pranayama has been one of the game changers for me. It is a powerful, transformative tool that must be practiced with consistency, intelligence, and patience. In 2002, I started a *pranayama* practice. Rodney had told me I should dedicate myself to it daily or drop it altogether—that I needed to take it seriously, because it isn't something that you just dabble in. He recommended I set a timer and practice only ten minutes a day for the first year. I'd get high off *pranayama*, seduced into spending a long time with it on some days and almost no time on other days. I also skipped right to the advanced practices of breath retention. I became irritated and aggressive and developed ringing in my ears. When you force *pranayama* before you're ready, it can be dangerous because you're dealing directly with the nervous system. Rodney had warned me about this and he strongly encouraged me to back up and simply watch my breath for a few months instead of manipulating it. I started back to my *pranayama* practice slowly and more mindfully.

There's a story about Mr. Iyengar's daughter, Dr. Geeta S. Iyengar. She went to her father and said, "Father, I want to learn *pranayama*." His response was, "Go and practice *shavasana* for ten years. Then come back to me. If you have mastered *shavasana*, I will teach you *pranayama*." Relaxation is the key.

My fifties have been about accepting that I'm enough. If I'm sad, I have the courage to cry. If I think something is funny, I laugh without control. Last fall I got a call asking me to give a talk about health and body image to young models during Fashion Week in New York. There would be media at the event, and the other speakers would be well-known experts in the health and wellness field. For an instant, I felt that reactive tug of *Why should they listen to me?* But then I told myself, "All I can do is talk honestly about what I know to be true."

At the event, I looked out into the audience and saw a hundred versions of myself thirty-five years ago. I told the young models that in a world based on looks, competition, and the seesaw of hope and disappointment, spending time in *shavasana*—settling into a relaxed body with a focused mind and smooth breath—can be a lifeline that connects you to your inner world, to a peace that isn't dependent on the next booking. This internal relationship will translate into a deep and profound sense of love for who you are, beyond your obvious external beauty.

Today, my daily asana, *pranayama*, and meditation practices are more important to me than ever. Ironically what I spent years frantically searching for was never missing. Yoga isn't just about being able to put your feet on your head in Scorpion Pose (even though that can be fun). Yoga is the practice that brings me back to my essence. It's a dear and seasoned friend I count on in every circumstance—from the burying of my mother, to the trauma and disappointment of my seizures, to the pleasure of sitting in the hot tub with my husband, looking at the stars.

At fifty-five years old, I don't necessarily have the same musculature, flexibility, and endurance I once had, but I do know how to listen to my body and can usually give it what it needs: energy, calm, strength, flexibility, or cardio. Sometimes, it's just a good *shavasana* that is the key to balance.

I like the fluidity and ease a consistent yoga practice provides. I'm grateful for the mirror yoga gives me to see my ridiculousness; when I find myself wasting energy on trying to prove something or get external validation, I call myself on it. Do I still feel a little bad after a class if none of the students tell me it was great? I wish I could say no. But the feeling usually lasts only a few minutes before I let it go.

I love Rodney with less fear and fewer games than I thought possible in a romantic relationship. We speak the same language with and without words. Rodney supports me, encourages me, and, most important, he listens to what I have to say with deep consideration and respect, and I believe he feels the same support from me.

The only way to integrate my own story fully is to live in the present, authentically, with kindness and compassion. Guilt, blame, and lack of forgiveness are huge barriers to knowing you're enough. Love is greater than any obstacle. It doesn't mean the obstacles disappear—they just don't consume you.

Each day I try to use my yoga practice to shed a few more layers of protection that keep me separate from others and from my essential self. I try to keep it raw and real. I don't have all the answers, and I continue to look at what is possible. I'm inspired by the courage of Fiona Apple as she dances her honest dance. I aspire to be as brave as she is, and to show that kind of strength and vulnerability.

As courageous as I try to be, I couldn't have written this book while my mother was alive. She was too proud and too private, and it would have upset her that people might judge me or our family for some of the less savory experiences of my life. But even though she died in 2012, I still needed her blessing to go forward with the project. I had heard of a woman named June Brought in Woodstock, New York, who communicates through "Akashic Records" with the spirits of those who have passed. My fall women's retreat takes place nearby, so I made an appointment to see her. If there was a possibility to connect with Mom, I was in.

I met with June and explained that I needed my mother's permission to write about my life. She asked a few questions, then nodded and looked into the corner of the room and relayed my wishes to the spirit guides. It took some time, but apparently she reached my mom, who said, through June, "If I were still alive, it would break my heart. But from here, I can see how important it is for you to tell your story, and I know it will help others." She gave me her blessing.

Then, according to June, she started getting bossy about Dad's care—telling me that I'm not responsible for it and that she is visiting him in his sleep and teaching him new dance moves (which may be why he was spending so much time sleeping at that time). She said some other funny things that sounded just like her. Who knows if I was really hanging out with my mom in that room in Woodstock, but I felt I'd connected with her.

With my mom's blessing, I went to my dad and asked for his. He cleared his throat and said, "Honey, all that stuff you've been through has made you who you are—and who you are ain't half-bad. You have nothing to be ashamed of." He added, "I'm eighty-seven years old and I'm not buying green bananas anymore. I want to read your book, so you'd better hurry up."

✦   ✦   ✦

Each December I go through a ritual where I ask myself what new seed I want to plant in the form of a New Year's resolution. Should it be the same kind of resolution I've tried for the last few years, like stop eating sugar? (Those roots don't seem to want to deepen.) My resolution last year was to plant a maple tree in our front yard in honor of my mom. I was six months late in getting around to it, but we finally planted it last summer.

Rodney and I bought a beautiful green-leaf Japanese maple, which was Mom's favorite tree. I sat next to the hole that had been dug for it holding a rosary that I had bought for my mom in Ireland, and said the Hail Mary for her. It was a brilliant, beautiful summer day, and when I finished, I kissed the rosary. "Mom, I love you," I said, and dropped the rosary in the hole, among the roots. Rodney took some photos. When we downloaded them later, we saw something strange—a green spot on the rosary. As we zoomed in, we could scarcely believe what we were seeing: a tiny shamrock attached to the cross in several of the images. I can't explain it, but Mom must have been having fun with us. She was making an appearance as we gathered in her honor. Rodney freaked out; no one had used Photoshop, and he had no way to explain it. So he shrugged and said, "You damn Irish witches."

I feel my mom every morning as I look at the tree. I can feel the roots and the rosary intertwining and inching deeper into the earth as I whisper a Hail Mary.

I'll watch the leaves die this fall, sprout next spring, and repeat the cycle again and again.

Mom, I know the tears you shed for your maple tree were about being in touch with your genuine heart. I'm still the little girl curled up in the box watching you cry. But now I'm a mother, too, standing at my own window, observing a maple tree, and feeling my own heart. I know you're laughing and crying and doing the Irish jig with me as I navigate this wild and wonderful world. When we know we're enough, the world shows us her beauty. Thank God, yoga is my companion on this journey. Peace. Shanti, Shanti, Shanti.

Yoga Sequence: Final Relaxation

Shavasana is my favorite pose. I play with different kinds of setups in order to drop deeper into its magical mystery ride. I love to place weights on different parts of my body to expose habitual tension and ease restlessness. Mr. Iyengar once said, "The stresses of modern civilization are a strain on the nerves for which shavasana is the best antidote." I'm one of the people he was talking about: a notorious multitasker who has difficulty quieting her brain and gets tension headaches as a result.

My favorite *shavasana* is with a sandbag on my forehead. For the first minute or so, I watch the pause after the exhalation. Then I scan my body from head to toe, noticing any lingering tension. *Shavasana* is about leaving behind our worries and expectations and dropping into the unfolding moment. On some days, my body becomes so vast, wide, and deep there's no sense of burden at all.

Asana practice addresses the tension we hold in our "gross" body—our musculature and bones. In *shavasana*, we drop into the body's more subtle tensions and start to release them at a deeper level, perhaps to the point where we let go of our "small" selves, our personalities or identities. Often, it's that personal lens that distracts us from the beauty within.

Staying conscious and quiet is challenging; our habit is to act or at least tell a story with the mind. In *shavasana*, we ask for no distraction—we lie on our mats for several minutes and relax with what is. This is often a very intimate moment with ourselves, when we set down our weapons, armor, security blankets, and ego and come face-to-face with reality. In that moment, we fall in love.

There is deep relaxation in knowing you're enough, in knowing that deep in your psyche you're already significant—and no amount of success or failure is going to change that. It brings about ease. With ease, there is clarity. And with ease and clarity come acceptance, love, and compassion, rather than resistance, confusion, and judgment. Ultimately, we hope to experience *samadhi*, the eighth limb of yoga, the connection with our true selves and the interconnectedness with all things. Consciousness becomes like a transparent jewel and all who come into contact with you see their own beauty reflected. *Om mani padme hum*. Hail to the jewel which sits in the seat of the lotus. May our practice polish the jewel until it is transparent and we are truthfully reflected.

Choose any one of the following *shavasanas* and stay for 10 to 20 minutes, or practice a few and stay for 3 to 7 minutes in each.

Final Relaxation (1). Lie on your back with a 1-inch-high folded blanket under your head. Place a strap around the middle of your thighs to hold your legs parallel. Then place a 10-pound sandbag (or another weight) on the tops of your thighs close to your hips. Use an eye pillow, which calms the mind by stilling the eyes. You can cover yourself with a blanket to retain the heat of your body, unless that makes you uncomfortable. The blanket under the head is calming. (Mr. Iyengar said that the head should never be on a hard floor because it jars the nervous system.) The strap around the legs ensures there's no tug in the pelvis from too much internal or external rotation. It also keeps the breath even and creates containment in the pelvic floor. The weight on the tops of the thighs grounds the femur bones and frees the breath.

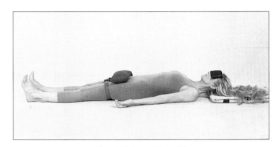

Final Relaxation (1)

Final Relaxation (2). Keep the legs strapped and place a bolster or a rolled-up blanket under your knees. This *shavasana* lengthens the lower spine and releases the muscles of the lower back.

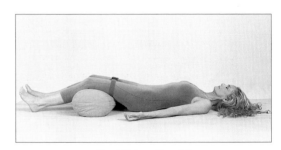

Final Relaxation (2)

Final Relaxation (3). Take the same pose as in (2), but this time remove the strap from your thighs, which will drop you into more familiar territory and may let you relax deeper.

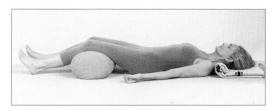

Final Relaxation (3)

Final Relaxation (4). Lie on your back and place your calves on a chair. Place a 10-pound sandbag on your shins close to your knees. This elongates the back by providing traction. The calves hold tension, so placing weights on them brings awareness to habitual holding, making it possible to release more completely.

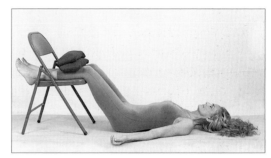

Final Relaxation (4)

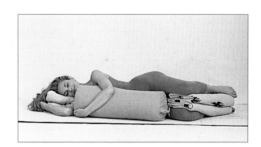

Final Relaxation (5)

Final Relaxation (5). Side-lying *shavasana* is very nurturing. Lie on your right side (or left side if pregnant), and place one blanket under your head and another between your legs from your knees to your feet. Then hug a bolster.

For each of these *shavasanas*, you can add an eye bag to create quietness to the eyes. When the eyes dart around, they agitate the brain. You can also put a block on the floor 2 inches above the crown of the head, place a sandbag on the block, and angle it so that the other end of the sandbag rests on your forehead. Make sure that the sandbag sits in a way that slightly pushes the skin of your forehead toward your nose. This is incredibly relaxing and calming for the mind, and good for headaches.

Meditation and Chanting. Chant *Om mani padme hum* 9 times. Then sit quietly for 5 minutes.

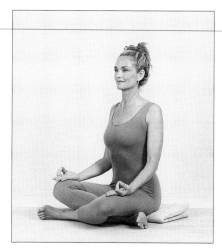

Meditation

It takes immense bravery to break a habit of thinking you aren't enough.

Using our yoga practice, we dig through all the pretense and protective layers, saying, "Nope, this isn't me; nope, this isn't me either," and we keep letting go until what we're left with is simple, real, and perfect. Stripped bare, we arrive at an open, raw state: This is who we are, and it is enough.

AFTERWORD

by Rodney Yee

Colleen Onora Marie Zello Kaehr Saidman Yee. You've already met the woman living between these pages. Now follow the name. Shall we start with the Irish gene that the name Colleen represents or Zello for the Italian? Or should we just say the mix turned out a drop-dead gorgeous woman who is intensely sensitive, head-shakingly intuitive, over-the-border brilliant, and ridiculously mischievous. The given middle name is Onora, which, along with Marie sets the Catholic confirmation into place. Follow the last three names and you'll realize I'm the third husband with the name that doesn't seem to match at all. But match we do. So please realize I am hopelessly possessed, obsessed, and in love with this wild, self-made woman. Here is my read of who she is, from the perspective of the pillow next to hers.

This yogi has a long arm of compassion for all who pass through her field of reach. Beauty, animal instinct, guilt, color, music, mother, wife, sister, daughter, and teacher are the words that immediately pop up. Her honesty is immediate and sometimes severe; it can result in the whiplash of guilt that arises from the possible result of her commentary. The essence of all of these characteristics is her genuine concern for the well-being of others.

She sees beauty and can cut through the overlay of BS that cloaks the natural core of love. She loves Sag Harbor, New York, because of the unbelievable light that illuminates the green fields that taper into the seaside. She loves the world of fashion and leaves the house every morning looking ready for a *Yoga Journal* cover in the most nonchalant way, never overdone. She sees the naked innocence of children and the sensuality of well-worn, aged faces. She may dislike the every-day superficial interchanges that make up too many dinner parties, but she loves the underbelly of people's stories. She teaches yoga to connect people to their real voices. So she loves the beauty of the skin and she loves the beauty of the soul. Everything in between she would rather leave on someone else's plate while we watch stupid TV.

There is an animal glint in her eye. She is more agile than a deer leaping fences, and her sense of smell for both the fragrance of flowers and the reek of insincerity is accurate and immediate. I kid her often about her smell capacity, and I'm afraid that someday my scent will gross her out. It didn't surprise me when she first told me about her boxing career because of her keen observation skills and her lightning-quick reflexes. We'll be at an important business meeting, and I'll see her disengage because she's already seen everyone's cards and the rest will bore her. For the most part, this animal instinct serves her well, but even the great yoga master Iyengar warned her about transitioning too fast.

When she turns on her heels and turns her back to you, it feels like you're on the dark side of the moon. Then her emotional boomerang of guilt kicks into high gear and she is waking up in the middle of the night, turning over and over her actions that may have caused you pain; brain raw from the conflict. Was it the Catholic Church and her mother that taught her the value of guilt? She often thinks I'm a jerk for not having enough of it. For better or for worse, this is part of her fingerprint, and in a twisted kind of way, it keeps me crazy about her.

We moved into a house in Sag Harbor we purchased together in 2007 after living for four years in her house in East Hampton. A local contractor had built and decorated the house in a lovely and typical Hamptons style, beautiful old barn floors with white walls and more white walls. It didn't take long for Colleen to paint each room orange, red, or gold. Color saturates her everyday life. She loves India, and when you walk into our yoga room, you smell the incense and see the vibrant colors of Calcutta. Up in our attic, her collection of dresses and shoes reflects these same aesthetics—clothes given to her by famous designers and those she buys make her current and alive. As she changes into her favorite sweatpants and my tee-shirt of the day, she sits in front of the computer to listen to samples of music that might catch her ear. It's the lyrics that tune her in. She is a teenager who looks underwhelmed by the present moment but then, out of the blue, you realize she has memorized all the words. Bob Dylan is her idol. I would give anything to be able to write her a love poem that moves her to that degree.

But of all things, what makes Colleen Colleen is her daughter, Rachel. Her need to be fully present for Rachel is huge. It is beautiful how she has taken in my children, Evan, Adesha, and JoJo, and made them her priorities also. She teaches us all how to be real with our kids in how completely herself she is around them. We often laugh at the seemingly inappropriate things she says, but then realize she is the only one willing to name the elephant in the room. The children adore her and turn to her before anyone else. She is quick to judge but has a compassionate touch.

As her husband, I sometimes wonder what the hell I'm doing with this woman. She has complete strangers proposing to her at airports. (I obviously wanted to understand jealousy and how it can be one of the worst obstacles to inner peace.) We challenge each other daily, but we are in physical contact 24/7. We feel complete when we are touching. She says she married me for my lips and my hands, go figure. Sometimes our closeness is hilarious; we often form the same thoughts and words simultaneously. So why me? Was it the Irish and the Chinese meeting at the Continental Divide in the building of the railroad or some reincarnation of past karmic debt? I don't need to know. All that is important is her breath upon my cheek.

◆　◆　◆

Why did she move to New York City, and why do we stay east when she values her family so much? This is her constant dilemma and indicates how much she loves New York and our wonderful yoga community in the Hamptons and in the city. She always knew she would be in New York. Colleen's mom and dad cherished walking around the city, and sometimes when Colleen and I have a moment off and we are strolling the avenues I get a glimpse of her lineage. New York, the crossroads for so many countries and the land of so many Romeo and Juliet romances, is home to the apple of my eye.

This woman turns heads and nearly breaks my neck daily, but the title that she has earned and is powerfully stepping into is that of yoga teacher. In this instance, I don't use this title lightly. I'm not talking about ten thousand hours or certificates of completion or some socially recognized position. I'm talking about an ordinary woman with the courage to dig deep, moment by moment, with compassion in her right hand and a sword in her left.

That Colleen is a gifted yoga teacher is an understatement. She registers every movement made by students in the room and gives insightful feedback and instruction. She creates unique and excellent sequencing, blending poses to un-lock difficult bindings that keep us from ease and freedom. Her struggles as a human being have helped her develop compassion for others—and to that point, she'll stay up at night practicing sequences that will help others with their predic-aments. Her intuition leads her to instructions that are cutting and profound. For example, she has a student who practices so precisely and intelligently that she can sometimes squeeze the life out of a pose. Colleen recognized her need for perfec-tion and blurted out, "Barbara, stop making your bed in the morning." Everyone in the room understood immediately what she was saying—the perfect correction for the perfectionist—and cracked up. Barbara stopped making her bed.

Her deep rapport with women makes her a leader and mentor for other women in finding their voices and their inherent strength. Women of all ages gravitate to her openness, genuineness, and nonjudgmental mind. When you show up at Yoga Shanti, Colleen is always the quintessential hostess, finding a spot and making you feel at home even if your yoga mat is halfway into the hall.

Right now, Colleen is letting go of the trappings of her past in order to be fierce in the present. She dares to be human in all of its colors, to stand naked in the white light and in the depth of darkness. She teaches because she falls and she gets back up and she wants to comfort us and tell us that we are okay when we do, too, and that we need to accept our wounds and our afflictions and get on with the day. We need to wonder and look and touch and hear and smell and taste again like a child, a beginner. She teaches because she has been to the darkest night of her soul and has returned with the knowledge that it could be even darker. She knows that she doesn't know, and there is no beauty in pretense. Colleen is learning it again in a different light and will teach us the nuance of this perspective through poetic lan-guage and creative yoga sequences.

Colleen writes this book to share a story that might make a difference, to share some yoga knowledge that might support you in just the right way on that heavy day when you need a lift. There was really no initial personal reason for her to make this monumental effort, but she was persuaded by her students, friends, and family to put down this story of internal and external obstacles and the peeling away of extraneous layers. Her map to her essential voice is a great inspiration for us all to get to work and continue to uncover ours. The woman I see in front of me is Colleen. No other name is needed.

ACKNOWLEDGMENTS

There are so many people who helped turn a hazy-crazy concept into a completed book. My agent, Esther Newberg, for starters, casually said to me one day after class, "Want to write a book?" I have never—*will* never—say no to Esther. My fear of and love for this woman—and my respect for her—is what got the book written. Esther is the most honest person I know: she only hugs people she loves, and she never says a word she doesn't mean. Once you win her over, there is no one kinder, softer, or more generous. To me, she's the quintessential yogi.

To my dad, Nick Zello, whose love of my mother taught me the meaning of love and dedication. To my talented, brilliant, crazy, and funny brothers, Mark, Joe, Nick, Ed, and John, who keep me humble and honest. To Peggy, my wonderful sister, whom I can always count on to say what I need to hear, just when I need to hear it. Peggy, thank you for always thinking I'm a good sister, even when I suck. I hope you know how special you are to me.

To all the yoga teachers who have taught me so much, and who continue to inspire me to get on my mat every day and continue my investigation. From my first teacher, Nancy Vinik, to Sharon Gannon and David Life at Jivamukti, to the gentle sage Richard Rosen, and to the love of my life, Rodney Yee.

To the Yoga Shanti posse, who keeps the ball rolling and the hive buzzing: Lisa Olsen, our manager (and much more), who welcomes every person who walks into the studio with kindness and compassion; my friends and teachers at Shanti—Padma Borrego, Trish Deitch, Steve Eaton, Heidi Michel Fokine, Stacy Haessler, Erika Halweil, Sarah Halweil, Kari Harendorf, Jenny Hudak, Leah Kinney, Joyce Englander Levy, Heather Lilleston, Stephanie Livaccari, Alex McLaughlin, Georgina McNiff, Kelly Morris, Hilary Offenberg, Eric Pettigrew, Brad Thompson, and Mitten Wainwright—who show up day after day and keep us on the cutting edge.

Thank you, Robby Stein—psychologist, friend, yogi, and local Sag Harbor philosopher/politician—for spending invaluable hours around our kitchen table, drinking tea and helping me see yoga teachings through the lens of Western psychology.

To Dawn Gallagher, for being my comrade in the world of modeling, for deciding to come with me to India to work with Mother Teresa, and for saving my life on the train.

Thank you to the careful readers and editors of this book, Trish Deitch and Carrie Schneider, who know sentence and story structure as well as they know asana; and Richard Rosen, who is one of the most brilliant and incisive yoga scholars and teachers of our time.

To my friend, student, teacher, and partner for the last fifteen years, Donna Karan. You are the most creative and generous person I know. You make me laugh when I need to laugh and cry when that is what is needed. I love you.

To the team at Atria Books: Judith Curr, Leslie Meredith, Donna Loffredo, Jennifer Weidman, Jessica Chin, Paul Dippolito, Patty Bashe, Sandi Mendelson, and Lisa Sciambre. You understood this book immediately and gave it the gift of your skill and creativity, shepherding it from a forty-page proposal to the book we hold in our hands.

To Rodney's and my kids: Rachel, Evan, Adesha, and JoJo, who wandered in and out of our house all year as I was writing, agonizing, procrastinating, giving up, then starting over . . . That they think my story is worth telling means the world to me. There are no better teachers than your kids!

Finally, to my best friend, lover, teacher, and husband, Rodney Yee. There has been no one more supportive during this project—or in my life. Rodney read every word. He directed all the yoga photos for this book, urging and demanding that I lift my chest more in Warrior I, and bend my knee deeper in Warrior II. Over the course of a year of nonstop writing, he cooked me and my cowriter, Susan Reed, omelets and tortillas—and it helps that he's the best damn barista (and tea maker) east of San Francisco. When I was frustrated and wanted to quit, he kept me going. When I suffered seizures, he held me and got me through them. He was, and is, an absolute rock. The writing of this book could have gone either way for Rodney and me, but it brought us closer. Rod, you are stuck with me. I adore you.

—Colleen Saidman Yee, Sag Harbor, New York, 2015

CREDITS

PHOTOGRAPHS

Cover by Zev Starr-Tambor; and pages 42, 60; back cover photos,
   all yoga sequence photos
Photos by Russell James: Pages ii, viii, xvi, 14, 118, 152, 180
Photos by Lynn Kohlman: Pages 28, 74, 104, 136, 204, 216
Photo by Robin Saidman: Page 90
Photos by Mark Zello: Pages v, 2

FASHION

Dress (cover) Colleen's wedding dress by Donna Karan
Colleen's yoga unitard by David Lee

Notes/Permissions

Page vii: "Kathe Kollwitz" by Muriel Rukeyser. Reprinted with permission of ICM Partners.

Page 29: *The Development of Personality; The Collected Works of C.G. Jung*, vol. 1. Copyright © 1954 by Bollingen Foundation, Inc., New York, N.Y. Reprinted with permission of Princeton University Press.

Page 43: Excerpt from "Forgiveness Is the Cash"; from the Penguin publication *The Gift: Poems by Hafiz*, by Daniel Ladinsky. Copyright © 1999 Daniel Ladinsky and used with his permission.

Page 61: Excerpt from *I Am That: Talks with Sri Nisargadatta Maharaj*. Copyright © 1973 Nisargadatta Maharaj. Reprinted with permission of The Acorn Press, Durham, N.C.

Page 75: Excerpt from "The Unbroken" by Rashani Réa. Copyright © Rashani Réa and used with her permission.

Page 91: "The Fruit of Silence Is Prayer"; copyright © Mother Teresa. Reprinted by permission of SLL/Sterling Lord Literistic, Inc.

Page 105: Excerpt from *Letters to a Young Poet* by Rainer Maria Rilke, translated by Stephen Mitchell. Translation copyright © 1984 by Stephen Mitchell. Used by permission of Random House, an imprint and division of Penguin Random House LLC. All rights reserved.

Page 153: Excerpt from "Empty," *Rumi: Bridge to the Soul* by Coleman Barks. Copyright © 2007 by Coleman Barks. Reprinted by permission of HarperCollins Publishers.

INDEX

About the Author

Colleen Saidman Yee is an internationally respected yoga teacher who has been teaching since 1999. For thirty years, she has been a top fashion model represented by Elite and Ford Models. Colleen opened her first studio, Yoga Shanti, in Sag Harbor, New York, and she and her husband, Rodney Yee, now have studios in New York City and Westhampton Beach, New York. With Donna Karan and Rodney, Colleen created and runs the Urban Zen Integrative Therapy Program, which is utilized in health-care facilities around the country. Colleen has been featured in *The New York Times*, *New York* magazine, *Vanity Fair*, and *O, The Oprah Magazine*, among many others, as well as in fifteen Gaiam yoga videos. Mother to a daughter and three stepchildren, Colleen teaches retreats, workshops, and conferences around the world but calls Sag Harbor her home.